Reviews

John Geyman has written an expert and highly readable account of the American health care system—how in the past 60 years it changed from a system devoted to caring for patients to one devoted to maximizing revenues—and he tells us clearly how to fix it.

> —Marcia Angell, M.D., former editor of *The New England Journal of Medicine* and author of *The Truth About Drug Companies: How They Deceive Us and What We Can Do About It*

John Geyman, one of America's most distinguished family doctors, has given us a masterful overview of what's wrong with our health care system and how to fix it. He supplements the daunting facts and figures with an engaging account of his life as a country doctor and medical leader.

> —David Himmelstein, M.D. and Steffie Woolhandler, M.D., both general internists, health policy experts, and professors of public health at the City University of New York

Dr. John Geyman describes the health care policy choices facing our new presidential administration, gently but firmly. As it has been since its passage in 2010, the Affordable Care Act stands squarely in the way. Dr. Geyman examined the options – repair, repeal, or replace – with the detail and documentation we expect from an expert observer and participant of American health care for five decades. Adding zest to this book is his memoir of how he evolved from geology major into an advocate for universal health care. The reader gains a greater understanding both of American health care and of one of the most highly respected veterans of our ongoing struggle to repair the world's most dysfunctional health care system.

> —Samuel Metz, M.D., adjunct associate professor of anesthesiology, Oregon Health and Science University, Portland

Dr. Geyman's description and analysis of the resultant hollowing out of the soul of medical care as the ongoing corporatization of medicine in America continues, and his prescription for change as seen through the lens of his 60 years long career, is invaluable. It is also a cautionary lesson about an even larger danger to America—that of capitalism-run-amok—a lesson that goes far beyond health care, and should be understood by anybody concerned about the soul of our country.

> —Phillip Caper, M.D., internist with long experience in health policy since the 1970s, and past chairman of the National Council on Health Planning and Development

In *Crisis in U.S. Health Care*, renowned medical reformer Dr. John Geyman offers a dazzling critique of U.S. medical practice and policy. The book begins with a well-documented, convincing historical study of how government programs, including Medicare and Medicaid, have supported the commercialization of American medicine, accompanied by enormous financial costs. The result has been to create an inequitable and unsustainable system in which, he argues, technology has been overvalued and individual patient care undervalued. Part 2 presents a parallel, moving autobiography of his own earlier service as a family physician in the Northwest and as a leader in the field of family medicine, which brings national debates down to earth. The central question here is what (and for whom) medicine should be for, over and above its status as a business. In the concluding section Geyman urges readers to dig into history, remember the principle of the common good, accept the social and economic benefits of a healthy society, and redefine the role of government to these ends. While there are no simple ways forward, Crisis provides an accessible, very readable and necessary jolt.

> —Rosemary A. Stevens, Ph.D., professor of history and sociology of science at Weil Cornell Medical College, leading medical historian, and author of many books on U.S. health care, including *The Public-Private Health Care State: Essays on the History of American Health Policy*

Our health care system is designed to serve first the market stake-holders and only secondarily the patients. John Geyman explains to us the history and flawed policy decisions that brought this about. As an icon in family medicine, both in patient care and in the academic arena, he adds his invaluable personal experiences to provide us with a crystal clear picture of what is wrong and what we can do about it—finally placing patients first, where they belong.

—Don McCanne, M.D., family physician, senior health policy fellow and past president of Physicians for a National Health Program (PNHP)

Geyman's latest book is at its best in portraying American medical care from the 1950s to the present through the lens of a well-informed, literate family doctor and teacher, one who knows more about American medical history than the pundits quoted on American television and on the pages of American newspapers.

—Theodore Marmor, Ph.D., professor emeritus of public policy and management at Yale University, author of *The Politics of Medicare*, coauthor of *Social Insurance: America's Neglected Heritage and Contested Future*, and member of the National Academy of Medicine

Dr. John Geyman's latest book is both a personal perspective and a well documented description of the change from the personal, professional physician-patient relationship of 60 years ago to our current medical system that is flawed by the overuse of technology, lack of follow-up care, and corporate greed. The author's conclusion: "Today's health care system, serving the corporate masters more than patients, is unfair, ineffective, inhumane for those left out, and unsustainable. Fundamental financing reform is inevitable, and is required sooner than later."

—John Raffensperger, M.D., professor emeritus of surgery, Northwestern University School of Medicine, Chicago, and author of *The Education of a Surgeon*

In all of American medicine there is no voice more authentic, more informed or more committed to the common good than that of Dr. John Geyman. In a career of over fifty years as practitioner in rural communities or as professor in the highest echelons of academic medicine, Dr. Geyman has championed care of the common man and woman, one and all. His current analysis and update of our medical system is both surgical and scholarly. Six years into the ACA, and literally on the eve of a new presidential administration, Geyman tells us the system is still broken and that it's breaking us. The cause (and its cure) are detailed herein with his usual no-nonsense clarity. He compares three pathways we might take to move medicine out from corporate greed and back to the common good.

—Rick Flinders, M.D., family physician and inpatient program director, Santa Rosa Family Medicine Residency, Sutter Santa Rosa Regional Hospital, Santa Rosa, CA

Also By John Geyman, M.D.

The Modern Family Doctor and Changing Medical Practice

Family Practice: Foundation of Changing Health Care

Family Practice: An International Perspective in Developed Countries (Co-Editor)

Evidence-Based Clinical Practice: Concepts and Approaches (Co-Editor)

Textbook of Rural Medicine (Co-Editor)

Health Care in America: Can Our Ailing System Be Healed?

The Corporate Transformation of Health Care: Can the Public Interest Still Be Served?

Falling Through the Safety Net: Americans Without Health Insurance

Shredding the Social Contract: The Privatization of Medicare

The Corrosion of Medicine: Can the Profession Reclaim its Moral Legacy?

Do Not Resuscitate: Why the Health Insurance Industry is Dying, and How We Must Replace It

Hijacked: The Road to Single Payer in the Aftermath of Stolen Health Care Reform

Breaking Point: How the Primary Care Crisis Endangers the Lives of Americans

The Cancer Generation: Baby Boomers Facing a Perfect Storm Second Edition

Health Care Wars: How Market Ideology and Corporate Power Are Killing Americans

Souls on a Walk: An Enduring Love Story Unbroken by Alzheimer's

How Obamacare is Unsustainable: Why We Need a Single-Payer Solution For All Americans

The Human Face of Obamacare: Promises vs. Reality and What Comes Next

Crisis in U.S. Health Care:
Corporate Power vs.
The Common Good

John Geyman, M.D.

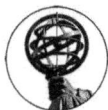

Copernicus Healthcare
Friday Harbor, Washington

Crisis in U.S. Health Care:
Corporate Power vs. The Common Good

John Geyman, M.D.

Copernicus Healthcare
Friday Harbor, WA

Ingram Spark Edition

Book design, cover and illustrations by W. Bruce Conway
Author photo by Anne Sheridan

softcover: ISBN 978-1-938218-22-4

Library of Congress Control Number: 2016960634

Copernicus Healthcare
34 Oak Hill Drive
Friday Harbor, WA 98250

www.copernicus-healthcare.org

Dedication

To Dr. Bill Reynolds, exemplary family physician and mentor over six decades, and thousands of other physicians in all specialties who have upheld the long and noble traditions of the medical profession and social justice despite the increasing commercialization of health care.

And to Gene, my wife of 56 years before her tragic death in 2012 from Alzheimer's disease, and to Emily, my wife today. Their encouragement and support through the years have made this book possible.

Contents
PART ONE
Reflections On System Changes Over the Last 60 Years

PART TWO

Then and Now: A Personal Perspective, 1956 to 2016

PART THREE

Today's Realities and the Future of U.S. Health Care

Tables, Figures and Pictures

Acknowledgements

As with my previous books, I am indebted to many for making this book possible. First, I have greatly appreciated the suggestions and comments by these colleagues:

- Mark Almberg, Director of Communications for Physicians for a National Health Program, Chicago, IL

- Marcia Angell, M.D., former editor of The New England Journal of Medicine and author of The Truth About Drug Companies: How They Deceive Us and What We Can Do About It

- Philip Caper, M.D., internist with long experience in national health policy work dating back to the early 1970s, past chairman of the National Council on Health Planning and Development, and founding member of the National Academy of Social Insurance

- Rick Flinders, M.D., family physician and inpatient program director, Santa Rosa Family Medicine Residency, Sutter Santa Rosa Regional Hospital, Santa Rosa, CA

- David Gimlett, M.D., family physician and former medical director of Inter Island Medical Center, Friday Harbor, WA

- David Himmelstein, M.D., general internist, health policy expert, and professor of public health at the City University of New York

- Theodore Marmor, Ph.D., professor emeritus of public policy and management at Yale University, author of The Politics of Medicare, co-author of Social Insurance: America's Neglected Heritage and Contested Future, and member of the National Academy of Medicine.

- Don McCanne, M.D., family physician, senior health policy fellow and past president of Physicians for a National Health Program (PNHP)

- Samuel Metz, M.D., adjunct associate professor of anesthesiology, Oregon Health and Science University, Portland, OR

- John Raffensperger, M.D., professor of surgery emeritus, Northwestern University School of Medicine, Chicago, and author of *The Education of a Surgeon*

- Rosemary A. Stevens, Ph.D., professor of history and sociology of science at Weil Cornell Medical College, leading medical historian, and author of many books on U.S. health care, including *The Public-Private Health Care State: Essays on the History of American Health Policy*

- Steffie Woolhandler, M.D., general internist, health policy expert, and professor of public health at the City University of New York

Thanks are also due to many investigative journalists, health professionals, and others for their probing reports on the evolution of our dysfunctional health care system. The work of many organizations has also been helpful in putting together an evidence-based picture of what has been happening in U.S. health care, including reports from the Centers for Medicare and Medicaid Services (CMS), the Center for National Health Program Studies, the Commonwealth Fund, the Congressional Budget Office (CBO), the U.S. Government Accountability Office (GAO), the Kaiser Family Foundation, the Office of Inspector General (OIG), the Organization for Economic Cooperation and Development (OECD), Public Citizen's Health Research Group, the U. S. Census Bureau, and the World Health Organization (WHO).

W. Bruce Conway, my colleague at Copernicus Healthcare, has once again done a great job with this project from start to finish, including book design of the cover and interior, typesetting, and conversion to ebook format. Carolyn Acheson of Edmonds, Washington, has created a useful, reader-friendly index.

Most of all, I am indebted to my wife, Emily, for her suggestions and constant encouragement through the entire process. She has read every part of the manuscript through its various iterations, bringing her eagle-eye to editing and proofing, while also helping with promotion of the book.

PREFACE

In 2015, I attended my Class Reunion from medical school, and with some surprise realized that I have been in medicine for 60 years. Those 60 years in American medicine—1956 to 2016— have been filled with enormous changes, of course including great progress, but also some losses.

Although I am reluctant to talk about my own involvement over these years, it does seem that I am in a position to share some useful insights that shed light on the positives and negatives in U.S. health care that may be helpful going forward. My perspectives have been formed, and informed, from a broad breadth of experience, including rural clinical practice as a family physician in the 1960s and 1990s, teaching and administration in three medical schools during the 1970s and 1980s, chairmanship of the Department of Family Medicine at the University of Washington for 14 years, editor of family medicine journals for 30 years, together with research and writing on our health care system for more than four decades.

There is widespread acknowledgment today that our current health care system is dysfunctional and broken, and I believe that we have reached a crisis point in U.S. health care. We need to better understand why this has come to pass if we are to avoid continuing in the same directions. The sixty years we will discuss have had many policy choices in how we finance and deliver care in this country. As we shall see, some have been positive, others problematic.

It is still a pervasive myth that U.S. health care is the best in the world—part of the American exceptionalism argument—but, as we will see, this is far from the case. Technology does not necessarily make things better, and we will look at how the traditional values of medicine as a profession have held up over the years.

How our health care system is organized and conducted should be above politics as a non-partisan issue, but we know that that is certainly not the case today nor has it been in earlier years. Despite ongoing national debates, we have still been unable to answer, as a society, even the most basic questions about health care, such as—Should we establish universal access to care for all Americans? Should health care be for-profit or not-for-profit? Is health care a right or a privilege based on ability to pay?

A word about my own politics. I was born into a Republican family, voted that way until 2000, but have become a progressive independent since then as it has become very clear to me that health care in this country needs fundamental reform. Our supposed system has become so complex and bureaucratic that it is difficult to cut through the detail to see how it could be reformed. Add political rhetoric unrelated to evidence, myths, and widespread disinformation fueled by forces dedicated to maintaining the status quo, and it becomes even more difficult to see the way forward.

All of my previous writing on health care has been based on evidence and experience, not ideology. That will be my goal here in discussing the many changes over these sixty years. I will try to use my personal journey and patient stories only to illustrate some parts of the changing landscape over these years. I will also try to avoid nostalgia, for we know that there is no perfect system, and that there is always a need for improvement in any time.

This book is organized in three parts. Part One includes reflections on system changes over sixty years. Part Two, then and now, gives my personal perspective from direct experience over these sixty years. In Part Three, today's realities are described, as are lessons that can be learned from the evolution of health care, three major alternatives for financing health care, and projections for future health care reform.

The results of the 2016 election cycle, which turned over the White House and both chambers of Congress to the Republicans, has placed our already broken health care system in continuing crisis. The first target for repeal or dismemberment, of course, is the 2010 Affordable Care Act (ACA), which provided 20 million Americans with insurance coverage, mostly through expansion of Medicaid in 31 states. Under the ACA's exchanges, 85 percent of new enrollees received government subsidies to help pay for that coverage. All of that is now in jeopardy, together with likely attempts by the GOP to further privatize Medicare and Medicaid. The so-called Republican "plan" for health care brings back such discredited features as consumer-directed health care, health savings accounts, high risk pools, selling insurance across state lines, and block grants to states giving them more latitude to tighten eligibility and cut benefits.

As the ongoing debates over the future of health care continue across the political spectrum, I hope this book is of use in cutting through the smoke and mirrors to the basic questions we still need to answer. Although the health care establishment may appear too imposing to be amenable to change, we have well documented evidence over the years that this most expensive system in the world compares poorly with other advanced industrialized countries in access, cost, quality, equity, and outcomes of care. We have had pro-market forces well entrenched for more than three decades that want to preserve deregulated markets that serve corporate interests more than patients and families. How to reverse that in the public interest is a matter of education and political will.

Come along with me on this 60-year journey as we try to make sense of all this.

—John Geyman, M.D.
Friday Harbor, WA
March 2017

PART ONE

Reflections on System Changes
Over the Last 60 Years

Government is instituted for the common good; for the protection, safety, prosperity and happiness of the people; and not for the profit, honor, or private interest of any one man, family or class of men. [1]

—John Adams, second president of the
United States and one of our founding fathers

---

1. Adams, as quoted by Hartmann, TA. A red privatization story.
The Progressive Populist, November 15, 2014, p. 11

CHAPTER 1

CORPORATIZATION AND CONSOLIDATION IN HEALTH CARE

Health care was a cottage industry 60 years ago, with most physicians in solo or small group practice, hospitals and nursing homes mostly small and independent with many not-for-profit, and private health insurers not yet in the business of medical underwriting in order to avoid coverage of sicker patients. Of course, it was not a perfect system, but health care was more accessible, at less relative cost, and with a more service-orientation to care than is the case today.

Corporatization and consolidation of U.S. health care has been a leading trend in its transformation over recent decades, in many ways not to the benefit of patients, as we shall see. Along the way, let's consider how John Adams' quote on the preceeding page relates to where we find ourselves today.

Some Historical Perspective

Voluntary health insurance, especially for the employed, grew steadily in the years following World War II, fueled in part by its tax-exempt status to employers. But since it was more available in larger, urban-located companies, it led to urban-rural inequities in insurance coverage. [1] In response to widespread concern over access to health care, Medicare and Medicaid legislation was enacted in 1965 as part of President Lyndon Johnson's Great Society program.

Both were opposed by the AMA, then considered the most powerful lobby in the capitol. [2] But millions of elderly and disadvantaged Americans gained access to health care that had been beyond their reach. Moreover, the effect of cost reimbursement and fee schedules for physicians in these two programs helped to reverse the nation's shortages of hospital beds and physicians, as well as deficits in medical education (through Medicare's funding of graduate medical education) and research. [3]

Corporate hospital chains were established within a few years after the passage of Medicare and Medicaid, together with many other health care corporations. As investor-owned facilities and services grew rapidly, Wall Street became enamored of the profits available in health care. Between 1965 and 1990, their corporate profits after taxes increased by more than 100 times, at a pace almost 20 times greater than profits for all U.S. corporations. [4]

The 1970s and 1980s were halcyon days for providers of health care, with most of the costs of physician and hospital services paid for by open-ended cost reimbursement and physician fee schedules. On the negative side, however, an ongoing period of health care inflation was ushered in that shifted the nation's overriding health priority from access in the 1960s to cost containment in the 1980s. [5]

By the 1980s, we had a surplus of physicians, especially in the non-primary care specialties, as well as of hospital beds. Health care costs were out of control, forcing the federal government and larger employers to take action. Both horizontal and vertical integration were starting to link health care systems as investor-owned corporate for-profit enterprises grew. By the mid-1980s, the eight largest investor-owned corporations together owned and operated 426 acute care hospitals, 102 psychiatric hospitals 272 long-term care units, 62 dialysis centers, 89 ambulatory care centers, and a number of other ambulatory and home health services. [6] In his landmark book in 1982, *The Social Transformation of American Medicine*, Paul Starr, professor of sociology at Princeton University, had this to say:

> *The rise of the corporate ethos in medical care is already one of the most significant consequences of the changing structure of medicalcare. It permeates voluntary hospitals, government agencies, and academic thought, as well as profit-making medical care organizations. Those who talked about "health care planning" in the 1970s now talk about "health care marketing". Everywhere one sees the growth of a kind of marketing mentality in health care. And, indeed, business school graduates are displacing graduates of public health schools, hospital administrators, and even doctors in the top echelons of medical care organizations. The organizational culture of medicine used to be dominated by the ideals of professionalism and voluntarism, which softened the underlying acquisitive activity. The restraint exercised by those ideals now grows weaker. The "health center" of one era is the "profit center" of the next.* [7]

Many physicians became more involved in group activity during the 1980s, including formation of independent practice associations (IPAs), while increasing aggregation was taking place among insurance carriers and health maintenance organizations (HMOs). In the early 1990s, Blue Cross and Blue Shield projected that 90 percent of benefits would be provided through managed care contracts by the year 2000. [8]

Pursuing their claims of cost containment and greater efficiencies through market discipline, investor-owned hospital chains invariably cut costs, especially by reducing nursing staff, thereby compromising quality of care while passing these "efficiencies" along as profits and dividends to shareholders. [9] Unprofitable services were often shut down, regardless of community need. [10]

Mergers and consolidation became common during the 1990s as hospitals struggled to survive in times of reduced reimbursement by payers. Some not-for-profit hospitals closed as others converted to for-profit status and some were acquired by investor-owned chains. Managed care was taking over the marketplace, with hospitals having to negotiate with HMOs for sources of patients and many physicians having to decide which HMO to join. Many physicians found it difficult to provide charity care, and some for-profit HMOs even forbade physicians from seeing non-paying patients. [11] Dramatic changes had occurred in relationships and influence between physicians, hospitals, HMOs, and insurers. What had been a pact between providers and insurers before 1970 had been broken as for-profit institutions and insurers gained power over physicians. (Table 1.1) [12]

As free-wheeling markets took over the health care system, Robert Kuttner, co-founder of *The American Prospect*, summarized the failures of market logic at the turn of the century this way:

> *In America, the over-reliance on market logic and market institutions is ruining the health care system. Market enthusiasts fail to tabulate all the costs of relying on market forces to allocate health care—the fragmentation, opportunism, asset rearranging, overhead, under-investment in public health, and the assault on norms of service and altruism. They assume either a degree of self-regulation that the health markets cannot generate, or far-sighted public supervision that contradicts the rest of their world*

view. Health care now consumes fully one-seventh of our entire national income. There is no realm of our mixed economy where markets yield more perverse results. [13]

Consolidation, Market Power, and Supposed Competition

What can we say about the market theory that consolidation with increased market power brings more economies of scale, brings down prices and costs, and adds to the value of services delivered? Actual experience in recent years shows that theory to be a total myth—larger market shares do *not* bring costs down or improve service, as these data points for four major health care industries show loud and clear.

TABLE 1.1
HISTORICAL OVERVIEW OF U.S. HEALTH CARE

1945–1970: Provider–insurer pact
Independent hospitals and small private practices
Many private insurers
Providers tended to dominate the insurers, especially in Blue Cross and Blue Shield
Purchasers (individuals, businesses, and, after 1965, government) had relatively little power
Reimbursements for providers were generous

The 1970s: Tensions develop
Purchasers (especially government) become concerned about costs of health care
Under pressure from purchasers, insurers begin to question generous reimbursements of providers

The 1980s: Revolt of the purchasers
Purchasers (business joining government) become very concerned with rising health care costs
Attempts are made to reduce health cost inflation through Medicare DRGs, fee schedules, capitated HMOs, and selective contracting

The 1990s: Breakup of the provider–insurer pact
Spurred by the purchasers, selective contracting spreads widely as a mechanism to reduce costs
Price competition is introduced
Large integrated health networks are formed
Large physician groups emerge
Insurance companies dominate many managed care markets
For-profit institutions increase in importance
Insurers gain increasing power over providers, creating conflict and ending the provider–insurer pact

Source: Bodenheimer, TS, Grumbach, K. *Understanding Health Policy: A Clinical Approach.* New York. *Lange Medical Books/McGraw Hill*, 2002, p. 189.

1. Insurance industry

The five largest health insurers have been on a buying spree, acquiring companies in health information technology, physician management, and other areas that give them more clout and market share to shape the delivery system in their favor. As an example, United HealthGroup, the $100 billion giant and largest insurer by revenue, sells technology to hospitals, distributes prescription drugs, manages clinical trials, and offers continuing medical education to physicians. In 2011, it purchased the management arm of Monarch HealthCare, an association based in Irvine, California with some 2,300 physicians in a number of specialties. [14] Its Optum division manages prescription drug plans, runs doctor offices, and analyzes health care data. [15] It has just announced plans to purchase Surgical Care Affiliates, a chain of outpatient surgery centers, with the deal to close in the first half of 2017. [16] Such acquisitions, however, do not make insurers more competitive or lower their costs. A 2010 report by the AMA found that 99 percent of more than 300 metropolitan areas tracked would be considered by the U.S. Department of Justice and Federal Trade Commission to have "highly concentrated" markets. [17] A 2010 report of a study that examined employer-sponsored health plans covering more than 10 million Americans between 1998 and 2006 found that "consolidation facilitates the exercise of monopsonistic power vis-a-vis physicians, whose absolute employment and relative earnings decline in its wake." [18]

2. Hospital Industry

The long-standing service-oriented hospital in the center of a community is a thing of the past. The more consolidated hospitals become in communities today, the more they hire physicians under productivity-based contracts that reward them for ordering more expensive tests and providing a higher volume of services. Costs to patients go in two ways—by doing more than is appropriate or necessary, and by hospitals charging facility fees, even when physicians are in their own offices but under contract to a hospital. [19] Many physicians have shifted their practices to specialty hospitals focused on only some well-reimbursed services, such as cardiac care and orthopedic surgery. These are for-profit and investor-owned (often by physicians practicing there), raising questions of conflicts of interest, as they give up other services, even including emergency rooms. In its periodic Community Tracking Study of 12 nationally representative communities across the country, the Center for Studying Health System Change concluded in 2006 that: "specialty hospitals are contributing to a medical arms race that is driving up costs without demonstrating clear quality advantages." [20]

3. Nursing Homes

Nursing homes are in a bigger corporate world than most of us may realize. A 2011 study found that 70 percent of the almost 16,000 nursing homes in the country are for-profit and 54 percent are controlled by corporate chains. The researchers of that study concluded that:

> *The chains have used strategies to maximize shareholder and investor value that include increasing Medicare revenues, occupancy rates, and company diversification, establishing multiple layers of corporate ownership, developing real estate investment trusts, and creating limited liability companies. These strategies enhance shareholder and investor profits, reduce corporate taxes, and reduce liability risk.* [21]

A follow-up study the next year documented worse quality of care in for-profit nursing home chains compared to their not-for-profit counterparts, with lower nurse staffing despite sicker patients and more serious deficiencies. [22]

4. Pharmaceutical Industry

Lurking below the radar is another dimension of this industry that has everything to do with costs, prices, choice and quality of service—pharmacy benefit managers (PBMs). They negotiate prices for drugs and the rates that pharmacies will be reimbursed, acting as middlemen between drug companies, pharmacies and their customers, which include insurers, employers and other groups. Here again we see big mergers and consolidation that bring huge market shares to this process. The 2011 merger of the two largest PBMs— Express Scripts and Medco Health Solutions Inc.—gave the new St. Louis-based firm, Express Scripts Holding Company, control over about one-third of the market in pharmacy benefits, almost four billion prescriptions each year. Representing pharmacists and drug stores, the National Association of Chain Drug Stores and the National Community Pharmacists Association worry that "the merged company will be too big to play fair, and will have immense power to unfairly dominate the market." [23]

Impacts on Physicians of These Changes

Corporatized health care in this country has had a profound and deleterious effect on physicians and how medicine is practiced today. These are some of the adverse impacts on physicians:

- Loss of professional sovereignty
- Loss of clinical autonomy
- Increased practice dissatisfaction and burnout
- Increased entrepreneurialism
- New conflicts of interest as employees of employers with whom they disagree on values
- Erosion of public trust

We will return to these impacts in more detail in Chapter 13.

What Impact Has the Affordable Care Act Had on Consolidated Markets?

The ACA was supposed to contain health care costs and make them more affordable. It has been a complete failure in that regard, partly due to its lack of price controls and partly because it has fueled a new merger frenzy among corporate giants in the medical-industrial complex. The CEOs of many companies fear being left behind and becoming prey for rivals. A number of billion-dollar deals have taken place as health insurers, hospitals, and drug companies have positioned themselves to profit from increased government spending on the ACA's exchanges, Medicare Advantage for baby boomers, and state Medicaid programs. The health care sector has led the way in mergers compared to the other four top sectors: oil and gas, technology, telecom, and real estate/property. [24] Gerald Kominski, director of the UCLA Center for Health Policy Research, summarized the ACA's impact this way:

> *The Affordable Care Act is driving this merger mania.*
> *There are billions of dollars pouring into the system, and*
> *it's money to buy insurance.* [25]

These examples show how extensive mergers have become in controlling large parts of the health care market:

Health Insurer Mergers

Over the last two years, the "Big Five" health insurers—Aetna, Anthem, Cigna, Humana, and UnitedHealth Group—have been attempting to merge to the "Big Three"—Anthem/Cigna, Aetna/Humana, and UnitedHealth Group. Should these mergers happen, these three insurance giants would control much of the market, with a combined membership of more than 132 million members. [26] But anti-trust enforcers are very concerned about harms to consumers from less competition. [27] A 2015 report by the Commonwealth Fund found that 97 percent of markets for private Medicare Advantage plans in U. S. counties were "highly concentrated," with little competition. [28] As a result of continued consolidation and withdrawal of the big insurers from unprofitable markets, it is projected that almost one-third of U.S. counties will have only one health insurer left on the ACA's exchanges. (Figure 1.1) [29] At this writing (early February 2017), it appears that federal judges will block both the Anthem/ Cigna and Aetna/Humana mergers in agreement with arguments by the U. S. Department of Justice. [30]

Hospital Mergers

As of 2014, the three largest for-profit hospitals in the U.S. were: Community Health Systems, based in Franklin, Tennessee with 191 hospitals; Hospital Corporation of America, based in Nashville, TN with 160 hospitals; and Tenet Healthcare Corp, based in Dallas, Texas with 72 hospitals. [31] As hospital systems expand, they typically buy up physician group practices in order to control large parts of medical practice in their areas. A 2014 study showed how hospital ownership of physician practices drives up prices and costs. [32] Martin Gaynor, director of the Federal Trade Commission's bureau of economics, makes this observation:

> *Hospitals that face less competition charge substantially higher prices. . . as much as 40 to 50 percent higher.*[33]

The Centers for Medicare and Medicaid Services, in an effort to make health care cheaper and more efficient, has recently mandated bundled payments for knee and hip replacements in certain cities. Though perhaps well intentioned, we can anticipate that this

FIGURE 1.1

ESTIMATED NUMBER OF EXCHANGE INSURERS IN 2017

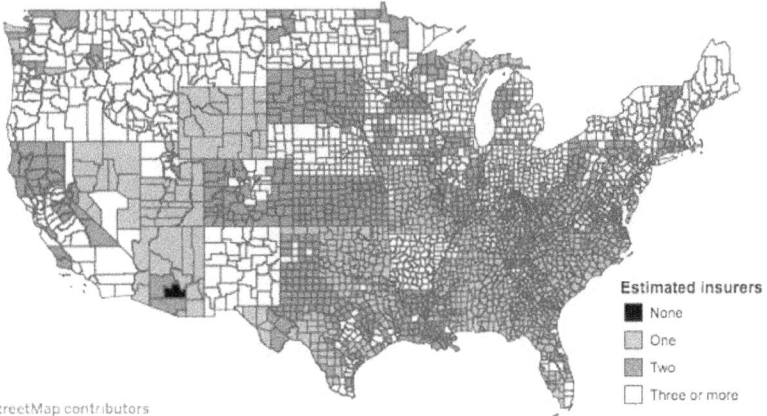

Estimated insurers
- None
- One
- Two
- Three or more

© OpenStreetMap contributors

Source: Kaiser Family Foundation, Preliminary Data on Insurer Exits and Entrances in 2017 Affordable Care Act Marketplaces, August 2016

will drive further mergers and consolidation as expanding hospital systems try to get in on the action. As David Friend, a managing director of BDO's Center for Healthcare Excellence and Innovation, says:

> *If you can get enough critical mass as part of these acquisitions, they'll need you and then you'll have a place in the new world. If you're too small, or too limited, you'll just become irrelevant and bypassed.* [34]

Drug and Medical Device Industry Mergers

2015 was a record year for mergers and acquisitions in the drug and biotech industries. Over the last ten years, the market value of biotech companies in the S & P 500 almost tripled to $594 billion.[35] Also in 2015, Walgreens Boots Alliance purchased Rite Aid, creating a chain of more than 12,000 U.S. pharmacies [36], and CVS acquired Omnicare to expand its reach into nursing homes. [37] In 2016,

Abbott Laboratories acquired St. Jude Medical Inc. in a $25 billion deal combining Abbott's stent business with St. Jude's pacemakers and implanted defibrillators. [38]

Concluding Comment

The main warring interests now are big hospital systems vs. insurers, with physicians and other health care professionals as employees and pawns in a big, profit-driven marketplace. No cost containment is in sight as free-wheeling consolidated corporatized markets prevail. The government is actually paying 64 percent of all U.S. health care costs, including subsidies to private insurers and qualified enrollees in the ACA's exchange policies, with minimal oversight and ineffective regulation. [39] We are paying almost double per capita for health care than in other advanced countries, enough to pay for universal health care for all Americans. Instead we are getting the most expensive system with access, cost, quality and equity problems as corporate interests rip us off.

We will return to that issue in PartThree of this book. But now we need to turn our attention in the next chapter to how health care has been increasingly privatized over the last three decades.

Endnotes:

1. Radovsky, SS. U.S. medical practice before Medicare and now—differences and consequences. *N Engl J Med* 332: 263-267, 1990.

2. Campion, FD. *The AMA and U.S. Health Policy since 1940.* Chicago. *Chicago Review Press*, 1984.

3. McNerney, WC. Rufus Reform award lecture. Big question for the Blues: Where to go from here? *Inquiry* (Summer) 33: 110-117, 1996.

4. U.S. Department of Commerce. The National Income and Product Accounts of the United States, 1929-1982: Statistical Tables, Table 6.21B.

5. Ginsberg, E. Ten encounters with the U.S. health sector, 1930-1999. *JAMA* 282: 1665-1668, 1999.

6. Gray, BH. (ed). *For-profit enterprise in health care.* Washington, D.C.: Institute of Medicine, *National Academy Press*, 1986.

7. Starr, P. *The Social Transformation of American Medicine.* New York. *Basic Books*, 1982, p. 448 .

8. Ibid # 3.

9. Woolhandler, S, Himmelstein, DU. Costs of care and administration at for-profit and other hospitals in the United States. *N Engl J Med* 336: 769, 1997.

10 Coye, MJ. The sale of Good Samaritan: A view from the trenches. *Health Affairs (Millwood)* 16 (2): 107, 1997.

11. Himmelstein, DU, Woolhandler, S. *Bleeding the Patient: The Consequences of Corporate Health Care.* Monroe, ME. *Common Courage Press,* 2001.

12. Bodenheimer, TS, Grumbach, K. *Understanding Health Policy: A Clinical Approach.* New York. *Lange Medical Books/McGraw Hill*, 2002, p. 189.

13. Kuttner, R. *Everything for Sale: The Virtues and Limits of Markets.* Chicago. *University of Chicago Press*, 1999, p. 140.

14. Mathews, AW. UnitedHealth buys California group of 2,300 doctors. *Wall Street Journal*, September 1, 2011.

15. Murphy, T. UnitedHealth looks beyond insurance to help fuel 4Q growth. *Associated Press*, January 17, 2017.

16. Abelson, R. UnitedHealth Group to buy outpatient surgery chain for $2.3 billion. *New York Times*, January 9, 2017.

17. Berry, E. Health plans extend their market dominance. *American Medical News*, March 8, 2010.

18. Dafny, L, Duggan, M, Ramanarayanan, S. Paying a premium on your premium? Consolidation in the U.S. health insurance industry. University of California at Los Angeles, 2010.

19. O'Malley, AS, Bond, AM, Berenson, RA. Rising hospital employment of physicians: better quality, higher costs? *Center for Studying Health System Change.* Issue Brief No. 136, August 2011.

20. Berenson, RA, Bazzoli, FGI, Au, M. Do specialty hospitals promote price competition? *Center for Studying Health System Change.* Issue Brief No. 103, January 2006.

21. Harrington, C, Hauser, C, Olney, B et al. Ownership, financing, and management strategies of the ten largest for-profit nursing home chains in the United States. *Intl J Health Services* 41 (4): 725-746, 2011.

22 Harrington, C, Olney, B, Carrillo, H et al. Nurse staffing and deficiencies in the largest for-profit nursing home chains and chains owned by private equity companies. *Health Services Research* 47 (1): 106-128, 2012.

23. Mathews, AW. Deal, combining two big rivals, will attract scrutiny. *Wall Street Journal,* July 22, 2011: B2.

24. Mattioli, D, Camilluca, D. Fear of losing out drives oil boom. *Wall Street Journal,* June 27, 2015: A1.

25. Terhune, C. Obamacare cash fuels healthcare merger mania. *Los Angeles Times,* July 2, 2015.

26. Mattioli, D, Hoffman, L, Mathews, AW. Anthem nears $48 billion Cigna deal. *Wall Street Journal*, July 23, 2015: A1.

27. Kendall, B, Mathews, AW. Health insurers face challenges to mergers. *Wall Street Journal*, July 20, 2016: B1.

28. Abelson, R. With mergers, concerns grow about private Medicare. *New York Times*, August 25, 2015.

27. Mathews, AW, Armour, S. Health plan choices shrink. *Wall Street Journal*, August 29, 2016: A1.

28. Top 10 U.S. for-profit hospital operators based on number of hospitals as of 2014. *The Statistics Portal* - htpp://www.statista.com/statistics/245010/top-us-for-profit-hospi...

29. Mathews, AW, Armour, S. Health plan choices shrink. *Wall Street Journal*, August 29, 2016: A1.

30. Kendall, B, Mathews, AW. Merger of Cigna, Anthem is blocked. *Wall Street Journal*, February 9, 2017: B1

31. Top 10 U. S. for-profit hospital operators based on number of hospitals as of 2014. *The Statistics Portal*
htpp://www.statista.com/statistics/245010/top-us-for-profit-hospi...

32. Baker, LC, Bundorf, MK, Kessler, DP. Vertical integration: Hospital ownership of physician practices is associated with higher prices and spending. *Health Affairs*, May 2014.

33. Baker, LC, Bundorf, MK, Kessler, DP. Vertical integration: Hospital ownership of physician practices is associated with higher prices and spending. *Health Affairs,* May 2014.

34. Picker, L. Health care companies see scale as the only way to compete. *New York Times,* April 28, 2016.

35. Walker, J, McGinty, T. Biotech births new fortunes. *Wall Street Journal*, June 25-26, 2016: A1.

36. UPDATE 5-Walgreens says will buy smaller drugstore rival Rite-Aid. *Market News*, October 27, 2015.

37. CVS Health and Omnicare sign definitive agreement for CVS Health to acquire Omnicare. *CVS Health*, May 21, 2015.

38. Walker, J, McGinty, T. Biotech births new fortunes. *Wall Street Journal*, June 25-26, 2016: A1.

39. Himmelstein, DU, Woolhandler, S. The current and projected taxpayer shares of U.S. health care costs. *American Journal of Public Health* online, January 21, 2016.

CHAPTER 2

INCREASING PRIVATIZATION
AND LACK OF ACCOUNTABILITY

Privatization was not in our vernacular 60 years ago. But it has become a driving force throughout our economy, especially since the 1980s, ranging from schools, water, and the military to health care. It is based on a myth that private is better, more efficient than public programs, and brings us more value.

In the last chapter, we saw how extensively corporate interests have increased their grip on much of the health care marketplace today. Privatization, of course, is closely related to that transformation. Here we will briefly trace its history, impacts on U.S. health care, and compare it with a public model of health care.

Historical Perspective of Increasing Privatization

In the ongoing debate in the 1950s and early 1960s over universal health insurance, as in earlier years, the medical, hospital and insurance industries strongly opposed any form of publicly financed health insurance. Insurers saw government-sponsored insurance as a threat to the private system and instead wanted the government to subsidize them in meeting the health care needs of the uninsured. At that time, they were discouraging older people from applying for insurance by charging them five to ten times as much for coverage as their younger counterparts. In the last stages of the debate over Medicare in the mid-1960s, the insurance and hospital industries began to see promising new markets.

The political battle over Medicare was intense as a conservative coalition, including the AMA, soundly defeated it in October 1964. It took a landslide election the next month to make its passage possible. When Lyndon Johnson became president, Democrats controlled both chambers in Congress, including a two to one majority in the House. Despite the continued strong opposition by the AMA, Medicare was enacted in July 1965 as a "three layer cake" that pulled together three different proposals—Medicare Part A (universal hospital coverage for the elderly), Medicare Part B (voluntary, supplemental physician coverage for the elderly), and Medicaid (an expansion of the Kerr-Mills federal-state program for indigent health care). This approach was intended to limit further future expansion of social insurance. [1]

In what became known as the "corporate compromise of 1965," all of the major players in the debate, even the AMA, were to profit immensely from Medicare as it passed with overwhelming bipartisan support in Congress—by votes of 307 to 116 in the House and by 70-24 in the Senate in July 1965. (Imagine such support today!). Private insurers did well by being relieved of their worst health risks—the elderly and the poor—allowing them to focus on younger, healthier, lower-risk people. They also gained having day-to-day administration of the program being contracted out to private providers and intermediaries, including Blue Cross, for claims processing, provider reimbursement, and auditing. Hospitals could anticipate many years of generous reimbursement of their costs of care for a previously disadvantaged population. The AMA gained a profitable "usual, customary and reasonable" reimbursement system that was flexible enough to allow wide variations in reimbursement for similar services from one part of the country to another. Physicians became well compensated for the care of many lower-income patients for whom they had previously rendered care on a charity basis. [2,3]

Traditional Medicare was conceived and first implemented as a social insurance program, not a social welfare program, in response to the private sector's failure to meet the needs of the elderly for health care. It provided, for the first time, a comprehensive set of health care benefits to all people age 65 and older. In so doing, it represented seven values and public policy concerns: (1) *financial security*; (2) *equity*; (3) *efficiency*; (4) *affordability over time*; (5) *political accountability*; (6) *political sustainability* ; and (7) *maximizing individual liberty.* [4]

The case can be made that most privatized health care has been made from public programs, especially from Medicare in earlier years and more recently, from Medicaid. During the Nixon administration in 1972, Social Security amendments were enacted authorizing Medicare to contract with private HMOs on a capitation basis, with the idea that participating plans would be subject to retrospective cost adjustments and constraints upon their profits. By 1979, just one plan had signed up. [5] That changed several years later, when Congress passed the Tax Equity and Fiscal Responsibility Act of 1982 (TEFRA), by which Medicare could contract with HMOs and pay them 95 percent of what traditional Medicare would pay for fee-for-service care in beneficiaries' county of residence. That launched a gaming system that would later end up with the government paying privatized Medicare *much more* than for traditional Medicare, with overpayments of about $283 billion between 1985 and 2008. [6]

In pursuit of their business model, private Medicare HMOs soon became expert at marketing their plans to healthier people and cherry-picking the market through favorable risk selection. That allowed them to keep their costs down, enroll healthier people, dis-enroll sicker people, and make a profit. A 1989 report by Mathematica Policy Research, under contract to the Health Care Financing Administration (HCFA), found that Medicare was paying 15-33 percent more for the care of beneficiaries in private Medicare HMOs than in the traditional fee-for-service program. [7] Nevertheless, the managed care industry continued to lobby for higher reimbursement, and many private HMOs withdrew from the market in the late 1980s, complaining of inadequate reimbursement.

Medicare managed care received a boost with the 1994 elections, when Republicans took control of both the House and Senate for the first time since 1954. As part of their Contract with America, they set out to transform Medicare from an "entitlement program" to one managed by the private sector, presumably with a lesser burden on government. House Speaker Newt Gingrich famously proclaimed: "If we can solve Medicare, I think we will govern for a generation." [8]

In an attempt to rein in overpayments to Medicare HMOs, the Balanced Budget Act of 1997 (BBA) reduced annual payment increases to 2 percent. That killed their hopes for a continuing market bonanza, so more Medicare HMOs exited the market. The main reason was their inability to contain their costs, especially of rising hospital rates and drug prices. [9]

The private sector soon fought back as the government tried to deal with a mass exodus of Medicare HMOs from the market. The Balanced Budget Refinement Act of 1999 (BBRA) gave Medicare + Choice plans new incentives, bonuses, and delayed the use of risk adjusters, but the industry wanted more. The next important bill for Medicare was the Medicare Prescription Drug, Improvement and Modernization Act of 2003 (MMA), which ended up a bonanza for the drug and insurance industries, continuing to ban price controls on prescription drugs, thereby assuring private health plans to receive $46 billion over the next ten years. [10]

Table 2.1 shows the main differences between privatized and traditional Medicare. [11]

The Affordable Care Act of 2010 (ACA) was intended to rein in health care costs and make them more affordable. It is singularly lacking, however, in any price controls or effective mechanisms to contain costs. Early on it was seen as a bonanza for corporate stakeholders in our market-based system. Tom Scully, former administrator of CMS in the George W. Bush administration, put it this way as the keynote speaker at a 2013 meeting of the Potomac Research Group, a Beltway firm that advises large investors on government policy:

> *Obamacare is not a government takeover of medicine. It is the privatization of health care. . . It's going to make some people very rich.* [12]

TABLE 2.1

COMPARATIVE FEATURES OF PRIVATIZED AND PUBLIC MEDICARE

PRIVATIZED MEDICARE	ORIGINAL MEDICARE
Experience-rated eligibility	Universal coverage
Managed competition	Social insurance as earned right
Defined contribution	Defined benefits
Segmented risk pool	Broad risk pool
Market pricing to risk	Administered prices
More volatile access & benefits	More reliable access & benefits
Increased cost sharing	Less cost sharing
Less accountability	Potential for more accountability
Less choice of provider & hospital	Full choice of provider & hospital
Less well distributed	Well distributed
Less efficiency, higher overhead	More efficiency, lower overhead

Source: Geyman, JP. *Shredding the Social Contract The Privatization of Medicare.* Monroe, ME. *Common Courage Press,* 2006, p.206

Today, 30 percent of Medicare's 55 million beneficiaries are in private Medicare plans, as well as more than one-half of 66 million people enrolled in Medicaid. [13] Figure 2.1 shows how the ACA failed to reduce overpayments to private Medicare plans, which amounted to more than $173 billion between 2008 and 2016. [14]

FIGURE 2.1

MEDICARE OVERPAYS PRIVATE PLANS

Total Overpayments 2008-2016: $173.7 billion

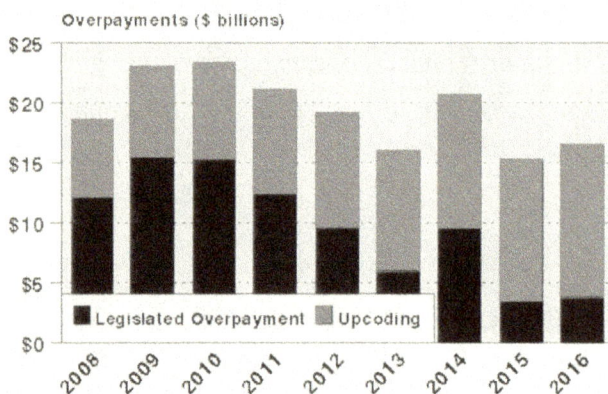

Source: MedPAC and Geruso and Layton, 2015

Source: PNHP Report 10/20/12 - based on data from MedPAC, Comonwealth Fund, Trivedi et al. Reprinted with permission.

There continues to be a prevailing myth, perpetuated by conservatives and corporate stakeholders, that we have a private health care system and need to fight the encroachment of the government in health care. The facts, however, are quite different. The government has been subsidizing private health care programs for a very long time. Two-thirds of our supposedly private health care system is paid for by the government—with our taxes! [15]

Figure 2.2 shows the extent of for-profit ownership of various parts of our health care system as of 2016.

FIGURE 2.2

EXTENT OF FOR-PROFIT OWNERSHIP, 2016

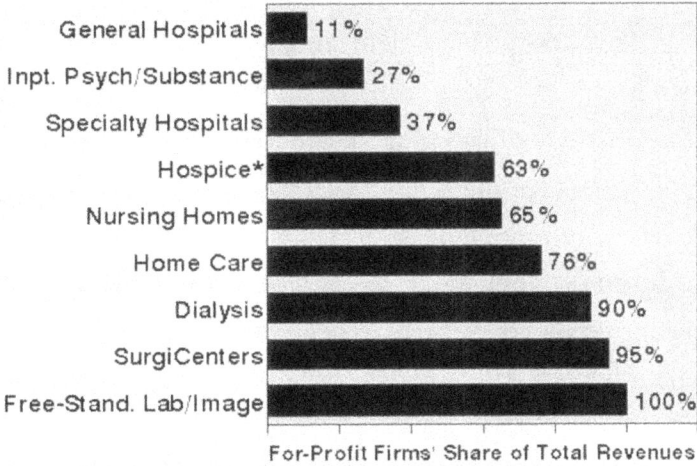

Category	For-Profit Firms' Share of Total Revenues
General Hospitals	11%
Inpt. Psych/Substance	27%
Specialty Hospitals	37%
Hospice*	63%
Nursing Homes	65%
Home Care	76%
Dialysis	90%
SurgiCenters	95%
Free-Stand. Lab/Image	100%

For-Profit Firms' Share of Total Revenues

Source: Commerce Department, Service Annual Survey 2016 or most recent available data for share of establishments.

We have evolved a system of large corporate welfare within our health care system—for the insurance, hospital, pharmaceutical and other industries—that feeds on public programs at the expense of taxpayers. As Ralph Nader, longtime consumer advocate, attorney and founder of Public Citizen, says:

> *Big corporations should not be allowed the myths of competitive, productive, efficient capitalism—unless they can prove it.* [16]

Lack of Accountability of Privatized Health Care

The following examples from across our market-based system illustrate how we get less and pay more for corporate stakeholders' profiteering:

Insurers

- Insurers have been gaming the ACA's risk-coding program, under which they are paid more by covering older and sicker enrollees, by overstating their health risks. [17]

- The Blue Cross Blue Shield Association has set up a new private health insurance exchange that will offer Blue Cross and Blue Shield Medicare Supplement Insurance (Medigap), Medicare Advantage plans, and Medicare Part D prescription drug coverage in more than 45 states and Washington, DC. This is designed to hasten the further privatization of Medicare by supporting employers' efforts to help retirees transition from group health benefits to individual private Medicare (Part C) coverage. [18]

- Medicaid insurers in New York State are cutting home-care hours for disabled patients, often without proper notice or legal justification. [19]

Medicare Advantage

- Medicare Advantage beneficiaries who need nursing home and home health care disproportionately leave it for traditional Medicare, raising questions about how well privatized Medicare plans serve sicker higher-cost Medicare beneficiaries. [20]

- Many patients on traditional Medicare are now surprised to find themselves automatically enrolled in private Medicare Advantage plans; CMS has actually secretly allowed these plans to enroll traditional Medicare patients without requiring them to opt in.[21,] but has recently suspended this policy.

- Federal audits of 37 Medicare Advantage plans have found overspending due to inflated risk scores, by overstating the severity of such medical conditions as diabetes and depression, for a majority of elderly patients treated. [22]

Medicare Part D vs. Medicaid

- Private insurers pay 69 percent more for prescription drugs under the Medicare Part D program than the costs of the same drugs under Medicaid, showing how negotiated prices by the government bring much more value than market dynamics. [23]

Privatized Medicaid

- Tennessee Medicaid plans, operated by BlueCross BlueShield of Tennessee, UnitedHealthcare, and Anthem, are typical of the poor service of private Medicaid plans, with inadequate physician networks, long waits for care, and denials of many treatments, even as the insurers pocket new profits. [24]

- Overpayments to private Medicaid managed care plans are endemic in more than 30 states, often involving unnecessary, duplicative payments to providers and calling for more scrutiny by auditors. [25]

- According to a recent investigation by the Office of Inspector General of the Department of Health and Human Services, fraud and abuse has been widespread in its Personal Care Services program, which provides elderly and disabled people non-medical assistance at home. [26]

*• Federal auditors recently found that private Medicaid insurers in Florida received $26 million over five years for coverage of dead people, mainly as a result of outdated information in state data bases and lack of coordination among different agencies. [27]

- Some states have received federal waivers to impose premiums and/or copays to Medicaid patients; this cost-sharing has been shown to result in disenrollment and decreased access to care. [28]

Hospitals

- Expanding hospital systems, facing less competition, charge much higher prices—by up to 40 to 50 percent. [29]

31

- Hospital charges vary widely across the country; one example: charges for a routine appendectomy in California have ranged from $1,500 to $182,955. [30]

For-profit, free-standing ERs

- The numbers of stand-alone ERs, unattached to hospitals, have been growing across the country, especially in more affluent areas; their charges are often four or five times higher than urgent care centers, and patients requiring hospitalization or surgery still need to be transported by ambulance to a regular hospital.[31]

Nursing homes

- Medicare is overpaying nursing homes for so-called "intensive therapy" at an increasing rate; Genesis HealthCare Corp., one of the largest nursing home chains, bills for this therapy seven times more frequently than it did in 2002. [32]

Hospice

- A 2013 investigation of hospice care by *The Washington Post* found that the number of for-profit hospices almost doubled from 2000 to 2013, with Medicare spending for that care increasing by five-fold; the investigation found the industry riddled with fraud and abuse, such as seeking out less sick patients who need less care and live longer, yielding higher profits, and offering their employees to recruit patients. [33]

Fraud

- Medical billing fraud is estimated to account for about 10 percent of all health care costs in this country, or about $270 billion a year. [34]

Lawrence Brown, professor of health policy and management at Columbia University, gives us this insight about the downsides of privatization in health care:

No other nation expects a private sector, little constrained by public rules on the size and terms of employer contributions, to carry so heavy a burden of coverage, and none asks private insurers to hold the line with providers (including specialists, uncommonly abundant in the United States) on prices outside a framework of public policies that guide the bargaining game. The first of these two grand exceptions largely accounts for the nation's high rates of un- and underinsurance; the latter mainly explains why America's health spending is so high by cross-national standards. [35]

Concluding Comments

Privatization, despite all its flaws, is increasing and threatens the survival of Medicare as we know it, as well as other service-oriented health care. There is a dangerous consensus among Republicans that the ACA should be repealed and replaced with an even more market-based system, and that Medicare should be further privatized and even phased out to the detriment of today's 55 million beneficiaries and seniors in the future. We will discuss these threats further in Part Three of this book.

We will have to learn, sooner than later, that markets and their business "ethic" are at war with the common good. They serve their corporate shareholders, not the public interest, and fail to meet any of the seven essential values established by traditional Medicare in 1965. We have enough money in this country to include all Americans in a single-payer system with universal coverage for comprehensive health care. The political and economic strength of the medical-industrial complex, however, stands in the way of that goal in our increasingly undemocratic post-Citizens United society.

This leads us to the next chapter—how increasing technology has impacted our changing health care system.

Endnotes:

1. Marmor, TR. *The Politics of Medicare*. Second edition, New York. *Aldine De Gruyter,* 2000, pp. 45-57.

2. Gordon, C. *Dead on Arrival: The Politics of Health Care in Twentieth Century America.* Princeton, NJ. *Princeton University Press*, 2003: 25-28.

3. Oberlander, J. *The Political Life of Medicare*. Chicago. The *University of Chicago Press,* 2003: 108-112.

4. National Academy of Social Insurance. *Medicare and the American Social Contract*. February 1999.

5. Oberlander, J. Managed care and Medicare reform. *J Health Policy Law* 595- 598, 1997.

6. Trivedi, AN, Gribla, RC, Jiang, L et al. Duplicate federal payments to dual enrollees in Medicare Advantage plans and the Veterans Affairs Health Care System. *JAMA* 308 (1): 67-72, 2012.

7. General Accounting Office (GAO). Medicare: Reasonableness of Health Maintenance Organization Payments Not Assured. GAO/HRD-89-41. Washington, D.C.: Government Printing Office, 1989.

8. Smith, DG. *Entitlement Politics: Medicare and Medicaid 1995-2001*. New York. *Aldine de Gruyter*, 2002: 71, citing Congressional Quarterly Almanac, 1995, p. 73.

9. Berenson, RA. Medicare + Choice: doubling or disappearing? *Health Affairs Web Exclusive*, November 28, 2001.

10. Pear, R. Medicare actuary gives wanted data to Congress. *New York Times*, March 20, 2004: A8.

11. Geyman, JP. *Shredding the Social Contract: The Privatization of Medicare*. Monroe, ME. *Common Courage Press*, 2006, p. 206.

12. Scully, T. As cited by Davidson, A. The President wants you to get rich on Obamacare. *The New York Times Magazine*, October 13, 2013.

13. Pear, R. As Medicare and Medicaid turn 50, use of private health plans surges. *New York Times*, July 30, 2015: A 12.

14. Geruso, M, Layton, T. Upcoding inflates Medicare costs in excess of $2 billion annually. *UT News*, University of Texas at Austin, June 18, 2015

15. Himmelstein, DU, Woolhandler, S. The current and projected taxpayer shares of U.S. health costs. *Amer J Public Health* on line, January 21, 2016.

16. Nader, R. The myths of big corporate capitalism. In the Public Interest. *The Progressive Populist*, August 15, 2015: 19.

17. Potter, W. Health insurers working the system to pad their profits. Center for Public Integrity. August 15, 2015.

18. Blue Cross and Blue Shield companies to launch retiree health insurance exchange. BlueCross and BlueShield Association, April 24, 2015.

19. Bernstein, N. Insurance groups in New York improperly cut home-care hours for disabled patients, report shows. *New York Times*, July 20, 2016.

20. Rahman, M, Keohane, L, Trivedi, AN et al. High-cost patients had substantial rates of leaving Medicare Advantage and joining traditional Medicare. *Health Affairs* 34 (10): 1675-1682, October 2015.

21. Jaffe, S. Some seniors surprised to be automatically enrolled in Medicare Advantage Plans. *Kaiser Health News*, July 27, 2016.

22. Schulte, F. Audits of some Medicare Advantage plans reveal pervasive overcharging. NPR Now KPLU, August 29, 2016.

23. Comparison of DOD, Medicaid, and Medicare Part D retail reimbursement prices. United States Government Accountability Office (GAO), June 2014.

24. Himmelstein, DU, Woolhandler, S. The post-launch problem: the Affordable Care Act's persistently high administrative costs. *Health Affairs Blog*, May 27, 2015.

25. Herman, B. Medicaid's unmanaged managed care. *Modern Healthcare*, April 30, 2016.

26. Bailey, M. Seniors suffer amid widespread fraud by Medicaid caretakers. Kaiser Health News, November 7, 2016.

27. Chang, D. Florida paid Medicaid insurers $26 million to cover dead people, report says. Miami Herald, December 13, 2016.

28. Levey, N. Four largest states have sharp disparities in access to health care. *Los Angeles Times*, April 10, 2015.

29. Pear, R. F.T.C. wary of mergers by hospitals. *New York Times*, September 17, 2014.

30. Rabin, RC. Wide variation in hospital charges for blood tests called 'irrational.' Capsules. *Kaiser Health News*, August 15, 2014.

31. Olinger, D. Confusion about free-standing ER brings Colorado mom $5,000 bill. *The Denver Post*, October 31, 2015.

32. Weaver, C, Matthews, AW, McGinty, T. How Medicare rewards copious nursing home therapy. *Wall Street Journal*, August 15, 2015.

33. McCauley, L. Investigation reveals rampant fraud by privatized hospice groups. *Common Dreams*, December 17, 2013.

34. Buchheit, P. Private health care as an act of terrorism. *Common Dreams*, July 20, 2015.

35. Brown, LD. In Stevens, RA, Rosenberg, CE, Burns, LR (eds) *History and Health*

Policy in the United States: Putting the Past Back In. New Brunswick, NJ. *Rutgers University Press*, 2006: 46.

CHAPTER 3

INCREASING TECHNOLOGY

The last 90 years, and especially the last 70 years since the end of World War II, have completely transformed health care in the U.S. as a result of technological innovation and change. Here we will briefly summarize this history, consider the benefits vs. problems of these advances, and ask to what extent they are managed in the public interest.

Some Historical Perspective

Almost all of today's approaches to the diagnosis and treatment of disease were unknown in 1950. [1] The 1950s saw the start of fiber-optic endoscopy, the first use of hearing aids with transistors, early use of computers, and the first randomized clinical trials. Among prescription drugs, 75 percent of the top-selling drugs in 1972 were not in that group just 15 years later. [2] The first CT scanner appeared in the 1970s and MRIs became widely used in the 1980s. Minimally invasive surgical techniques have flourished in recent decades, ranging from laparoscopic abdominal surgery to cardiac surgery. Other advances in more recent years include robotic devices for computer-assisted surgery, sequencing of the human genome, regenerative medicine, and "precision medicine" through pharmacogenomics (PGx). Table 3.1 shows the chronology of some of these technological advances since the 1920s. [3]

It is remarkable how quickly new procedures or techniques have been assimilated in our health care system. As examples, liver

CHRONOLOGY OF TECHNICAL ADVANCES IN MEDICAL CARE

1920

First use of x-rays in diagnosis

1930

Discovery of electron microscopes

Sulfa drugs developed

Start of blood bank

Early use of insulin for diabetes mellitus

1940

Penicillin a breakthrough for many infectious diseases

Modern anesthesia emerged with muscle relaxants

Genetics linked to biochemistry

DNA molecule described

Nitrogen mustard—the first chemotherapy agent for cancer (lymphoma)

1950

Start of fiberoptic endoscopy

First hearing aids with transistors

Early use of computers

First use of tricyclic antidepressants

Advances in prosthetic limbs

Increased use of radiation therapy for cancer

Increasing use of cortisone and derivatives

Increasing recognition of genetic basis of disease

First randomized clinical trials

1960

Kidney transplants in growing use

Immunology established as active clinical field

First use of ultrasound

First laser surgery

Biological psychiatry and emergence of psychoactive drugs

Start of coronary bypass surgery

First hip replacements

First cardiac pacemaker

Oral contraceptives in common use

Renal dialysis for chronic renal failure

1970

First CT scanner

First use of angioplasty for coronary artery disease

Emergence of genetic engineering

1980

MRIs become widely used

Smallpox eradicated

Growing use of recombinant vaccines and drugs

Liver transplantation

1990

Peptic ulcer tied to *Helicobacter pylori*

Progress with antiretroviral drugs

Introduction of laser refractive eye surgery

Other organ transplantation

Genotypes identified for some breast and colon cancer

2000

FDA approval of robotic device for computer assisted surgery

2010

Genetically targeted cancer drugs

Increasing use of robotic surgery

3-D printing for pre-surgery planning and other uses

transplants increased from 26 in 1981 to more than 1,100 just six years later (1); by 1996, 60,000 heart valve replacements were performed each year, as well as 150,000 knee prostheses. [4]

Medical technology encompasses a broader spectrum than we might realize on first thought. Some 20 years ago, for example, the New Technology Committee of Kaiser Permanente divided new procedures and technology into these four categories:

"1. New procedures that involve new and expensive equipment (e.g. lithotripsy),
2. New procedures that do not involve new equipment or drugs (e.g. in vitro fertilization),
3. New drugs (e.g. genetically engineered drugs, very expensive drugs, such as Ceredase), and
4. New technologies developed for life-threatening diseases (e.g. liver or heart transplantation)." [5]

Lewis Thomas, as a leading analyst of medical progress, described in 1975 these three useful ways of looking at medical technologies:

1. *Nontechnology*—non-curative care for patients with advanced diseases whose natural history cannot be changed (e.g. intractable cancer, advanced cirrhosis).
2. *Halfway technology*—also care that is non-curative but may delay death (e.g. liver or heart transplants).
3. *High technology*—curative treatment or effective prevention techniques (e.g. polio vaccination). [6]

Unfortunately, most of our technological advances are of the halfway non-curative type. Since they are often overused at great expense, this presents society a challenging task to manage their adoption in a cost-effective way.

Technology as a Double-Edged Sword

There is no question that many advances have been of great benefit to individual patients and society, such as replacement of hips and knees, coronary bypass surgery, and cataract surgery with prescription intra-ocular lens replacement. But there are downsides as well, as illustrated by the not widely known adverse events in robotic surgery. Between 2007 and 2013, more than 1.74 million robotic procedures were performed in this country, most commonly in gynecology and urology, with 144 deaths (1.4 percent), 1,391 patient injuries (13.1 percent), and more than 8,000 device malfunctions (75.9 percent). Device and instrument malfunctions were quite common, and in 10 percent of the procedures, the procedure had to be interrupted to re-start the system, convert to non-robotic techniques, or reschedule it to a later time. [7]

At the macro level, Drs. Elliott Fisher and Gilbert Welch, based at the Center for the Evaluative Clinical Sciences at Dartmouth Medical School, have called attention to the unintended consequences in the growth of medical care by way of "the law of diminishing returns." (Figure 3.1) They follow this up by showing us the various pathways by which more medical care may lead to harm, as shown in Figure 3.2. [8]

It has become very common that incidental findings in CT scans, MRIs and other imaging tests lead to inappropriate, expensive and sometimes harmful further testing. Radiologists may feel trapped legally for fear of medical legal liability if further testing is not done. The frequency of incidental findings, often clinically insignificant, is higher than we might imagine—40 to 70 percent of CT scans of the abdomen and 40 percent for CT scans of the lumbar spine. [9]

In addition to the growth of new technologies, there are two other main drivers of transformational change—medicalization of

FIGURE 3.1

THE LAW OF DIMINISHING RETURNS

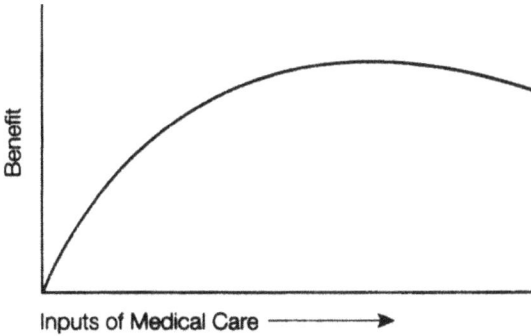

The first unit of input provides substantial benefits (imagine the first physician in a community), while additional units provide declining additional benefits (imagine the thousandth physician). Eventually, increasing inputs lead to no additional benefit (the "flat of the curve"). At some point, in theory, additional inputs lead to harm.

Source: Fisher, ES, Welch, HG. Avoiding the unintended consequences of growth in medical care: How might more be worse? *JAMA* 281:446-453, 1999. Reprinted with permission.

FIGURE 3.2

PATHWAYS BY WHICH MORE MEDICAL CARE MAY LEAD TO HARM

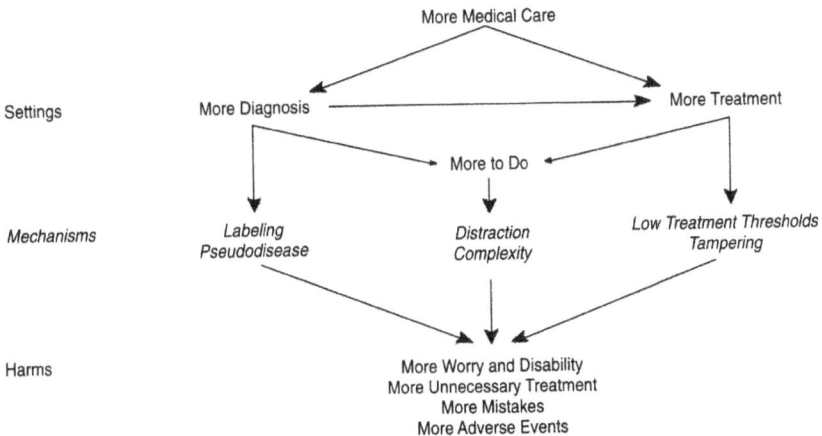

Source: Fisher, ES, Welch, HG. Avoiding the unintended consequences of growth in medical care: How might more be worse? *JAMA* 281:446-453, 1999. Reprinted with permission.

preventive and therapeutic services and promotion leading to increased demand for services, whether necessary or not.

The boundaries of health care have expanded enormously in the last 60 years. Some have taken place gradually as socio-cultural changes, such as the rapid growth of aesthetic medicine for cosmetic skin care. [10] *New diagnostic tools* further add to boundary expansion of health care, such as MRI scanning that now finds "abnormalities" in completely asymptomatic people; one study found that one-half of young adults were found to have lumbar disk bulge without any back pain. [11] The widespread adoption of fetal monitoring led to more aggressive management of labor and a marked increase in the number of Caesarian sections with little evidence of improved outcomes.

Changing definitions of existing diseases also contributes to expanded health care, as illustrated by the prevalence of hypercholesterolemia increasing by 86 percent after the threshold level for "disease" was lowered from 240 mg/dl to 200 mg/dl. [12] *Definition of new diseases* is still another powerful boundary expander, such as by promotion of the blockbuster drug Viagra for erectile dysfunction and the pharmaceutical industry's efforts to widely define and treat female sexual dysfunction. [13]

The above drivers of expanded health care are further multiplied by vigorous promotion of products and procedures by providers and suppliers. Direct-to-consumer advertising of drugs has been a large marketing strategy for many years, and has been joined by direct-to-consumer advertising of surgical procedures, such as for joint replacement. Some of these marketing strategies have become so subtle as to not be seen by consumers as advertising, such as through "health newsletters" as point-of-purchase ads wrapped into warning labels given to patients picking up their prescriptions. [14]

As early as 1988, Harvard psychiatrist Arthur Barsky described the marketing of corporate stakeholders in our medical-industrial complex in these words which, unfortunately, are still right on target:

> *Health is industrialized and commercialized in a fashion that enhances many people's dissatisfaction with their health. Advertisers, manufacturers, advocacy groups, and proprietary health care corporations promote the myth that good health can be purchased; they market products and services that purport to deliver the consumer into the promised land of wellness. A giant medical-industrial complex has arisen, composed initially of for-profit health care corporations, such as free-standing ambulatory surgery centers, free-standing diagnostic laboratories, home health care services, and of course proprietary hospitals. But the market is so lucrative that the products of the medical-industrial complex now range all the way from do-it-yourself diagnostic kits to "lite" foods, from tooth polish to eye drops, from health magazines to Medic-Alert bracelets, from exercise machines to fat farms.* [15]

Can Health Care Technology Be Managed in the Public Interest?

The pressures are immense, from various quarters, for early adoption of new technologies even before their benefits or cost-effectiveness have been established by credible science. Direct-to-consumer advertising of drugs and other services is a powerful way of building new markets. This advertising is often misleading or deceptive, and may be done through video news releases (VNRs) for products without FDA approval. [16]

Two examples from industry give us a sense of how strong and subtle the pressures can be from manufacturers to adopt new technologies, mostly below the radar of public awareness. The *drug in-*

43

dustry has a long history of delayed or inaccurate reporting of risks and adverse outcomes [17], commissioning ghost writers to write articles promoting their products without regard to their risks [18], publishing favorable research results while suppressing publication of negative results [19], manipulating the process of clinical guideline development for marketing purposes [20], and sharing non-public scientific data with selected Wall Street analysts while calling on them not to share the information. [21] Phase IV drug trials, also known as "seeding trials," are typically conducted by drug companies' *marketing* departments. These "studies" have no scientific rigor or credibility and lack federal human subject protections. They can also be dangerous for patients, as happened when 11 patients died and 73 others had serious adverse events (none of which were publicized) during a twelve-year seeding trial of Pfizer's seizure drug, Neurontin. [22]

The *medical device industry* has a large market ranging from cardiac pacemakers and defibrillators to lasers, hip and knee replacements. When it comes to putting markets ahead of patient safety, this industry has a record similar to the pharmaceutical industry. One measure of its risks to public safety is the recall of more than 1,000 medical devices each year. [23] Manufacturers of medical devices often delay notification to the FDA about negative experiences with their products, continue marketing them beyond adverse reports, and seek protection from willing legislators. One example of such a delaying action involved Guidant's short-circuiting implantable heart defibrillators. [24] A more recent example was the defective all-metal ASR hip replacement, which the DePuy orthopedic division of Johnson & Johnson continued to market overseas and marketed a closely related implant in this country through a regulatory loophole not requiring evidence of safety or effectiveness. The company finally recalled these implants after failure rates continued to grow both in this country and abroad, resulting in the filing of some 5,000 lawsuits against the company. [25]

The political process is another less obvious factor that can lead to increasing medicalization of our society, as exemplified by state legislators mandating school screening of children for scoliosis in 26 states without evidence of effectiveness. [26] And of course, the connections between corporate stakeholders and government have been closely intertwined for many years through lobbying, deregulation, and a revolving door of leadership between government, regulators, and industry.

Once new technology is adopted, it can also be difficult to discontinue its use, even when later proven ineffective or even harmful. Enter the word *"de-innovate"*, the process whereby clinicians give up old practices. A recent journal article dealt with the challenge of overcoming resistance to de-innovation, as illustrated by the latest science-based recommendations to discontinue screening mammograms before age 50 and the use of PSA testing for prostate cancer. Both recommendations have been met by widespread skepticism by many physicians, patients, and some organizations despite the science that informed the changes. [27]

So, given all of these problems, we need to ask—what's been done to evaluate and regulate the adoption and use of medical technologies, and has it worked? Two national organizations were established in the 1970s—the Office of Technology Assessment (OTA) in 1975 and the National Center Health Care Technology (NCHCT) in 1978—but both were later abolished after a strong backlash from powerful vested interests, especially the medical devices industry and several medical professional societies. [28-30]

The FDA has long been handcuffed by political forces preventing comparative evaluations of competing technologies with a requirement for evidence of long-term outcomes. Moreover, over the years it has been underfunded, lacks sufficient authority, and is dependent on the industries it supposedly regulates through recurrent authorizations of user fees—a fox-in-the-henhouse situation. Examples abound of its lack of adequate oversight of health technologies. Here are just four:

- A 2008 study found that among 90 drugs approved by the FDA between 1998 and 2000, only 394 of 909 clinical trials were ever published in a peer-reviewed journal. [31]
- Johnson & Johnson's Gynecare Prolift mesh received expedited FDA approval as a less invasive treatment for pelvic organ prolapse, despite lack of clinical trials or demonstrated efficacy; problems followed, including treatment failures and deaths, and the Institute of Medicine called for more rigorous review of the FDA's approval process. [32]
- The FDA allowed expanded marketing of off-label cancer drugs in 2009 despite the lack of clinical evidence of their effectiveness. [33]
- A study of FDA-approved drugs subsequently withdrawn from the market between 1993 and 2010 found that unsafe drugs were prescribed more than 100 million times in the United States before being recalled from the market. [34]

Health care industries collectively spent $489 million on lobbying in 2014, about one-half of which was spent by the drug industry in its continuing effort to head off any attempts to control drug prices and to gain more rapid FDA approval based on weaker evidence. Gilead, which markets Sovaldi for the treatment of hepatitis C, hired 26 lobbyists to lobby successfully for FDA approval and payment by CMS for screening. (Sovaldi is the $1,000 a pill drug costing $84,000 for a full course of treatment). Conflicts of interest are common—many reviewers on FDA panels have close ties to industry and one-half of all health care lobbyists are former government officials. [35]

The harms that result from our weak regulatory process are obvious. Beyond the potentially preventable adverse events and even deaths resulting from drugs and procedures that should not have been approved, we end up paying more for unnecessary and inappropriate services of little value. As two examples of overuse of technology, despite the lack of evidence of benefit or approval by the FDA and the American College of Radiology, more than 30 million full-body CT scans are performed every year for screening purposes, posing a threat of potentially harmful radiation exposure. [36] Fetal ultrasounds are also greatly overused—more than 5 in 2014 per delivery, up by 92 percent since 2004, despite warnings by the American College of Obstetricians and Gynecologists that two should suffice in low-risk pregnancies. [37]

Concluding Comment

We can see that we have a long way to go to rein in advancing technologies in the public interest. Technology development leads to an arms race in expensive and lucrative products and procedures that raise critical issues of priorities and equity within our health care system. When resources are limited, as they are in the real world, how do we decide between heart transplants, which benefit only a few people with marginal outcomes, and public health or preventive measures that can benefit millions? And how can we decide whether and how to pay for genome testing for some cancers at a time when we have no idea about the potential costs and benefits down the road?

Health care technology is way ahead of our ability as a profession and society to deal with its future impacts, such as effectiveness and cost. We tend to adopt new technologies without asking the bigger questions, then are left with its consequences. Technological "advances" raise new and still largely unanswered questions, such as: what really works, who decides, are coverage decisions affordable and accountable, will everyone have access to necessary services or do we increase our multi-tiered system, and what is the role of government vs. markets? More importantly, of course, who is the system for—corporate stakeholders or patients and their families? These questions have economic, social, political and moral dimensions, as do their answers. In order to reach answers that are acceptable on medical, social, economic and moral grounds, we will need evidence-based science, leadership by health professionals and their organizations, an appropriate level of government regulation, responsible media, and a democratic process serving the common good. Standing in the way of that are trends in the health care marketplace that we discussed in the last two chapters.

Endnotes:

1. Weisbrod, BA. The nature of technological change: Incentives matter! In Committee on Technological Innovation in Medicine. Institute of Medicine, Gelijns, AC, Dawkins, HV (eds). *Adopting new medical technology. Medical Innovation at the crossroads,* vol 4. Washington, D.C., *National Academy Press,* 1994: 10.

2. Cleeton, D, Goepfrich, VT, Weisbrod, BA. The consumer price index for prescription drugs; dealing with technological change. Working paper, University of Wisconsin, Madison, Center for Health Economics and Law, 1998.

3. Updated from Geyman J.P. *Health Care in America: Can Our Ailing System Be Healed?* Boston. *Butterworth Heinemann,* 2002, p.16

4. Gorman, C, Siler, C. Transplants. *Time.* 1996 (Fall): 73.

5. Lairson, PD. Kaiser Permanente's new technology committee: Coverage decision making in a group model. Health maintenance organization. In Ibid # 1, 1994: 103-104.

6. Thomas, L. *The Lives of a Cell: Notes from a Biology Watcher*. New York. *Bantam Books*, 1975.

7. Alemzadeh, H, Iyer, RK, Kalbarczyk, Z et al. Adverse events in robotic surgery: a retrospective study of 14 years of FDA data. Cornell University Library, July 21, 2015.

8. Fisher, ES, Welch, HG. Avoiding the unintended consequences of growth in medical care: How might more be worse? *JAMA* 281: 446-453, 1999.

9. Lagnado, L. When a medical test leads to another, and another. *Wall Street Journal*, August 30, 2016: D1.

10. Manning, M. Anti-aging becomes big business. Doctors open medical spas around the country. *Tampa Bay Business Journal*, December 8, 2006: 33.

11. Jensen, MC, Brant-Zawadzki, MN, Obuchowski, N et al. Magnetic resonance imaging of the lumbar spine in people without back pain. *N Engl J Med* 331: 669-73, 1994.

12. Schwartz, LM, Wolosin, S. Changing disease definitions: implications for disease prevalence. Analysis of the Third National Health and Nutrition Examination Survey. *Eff Clin Pract* 2 (2): 26-35, 1999.

13. Moynihan, R. The making of a disease: Female sexual dysfunction. *BMJ* 326: 45, 2003.

14. Armstrong, D, Zimmerman, A. Drug makers find new way to push pills. *Wall Street Journal*, June 14, 2002: B1.

15. Barsky, AJ. The paradox of health. *N Engl J Med* 318: 414-418, 1988.

16. Foley, KE. Ethics and Sigma are in 'VNR cartel.' *O'Dwyer's PR Services Report*, April 1993, p. 13.

17. Wolfe, SM (ed) Sleight-of-hand. Merck contemplated Vioxx reformulation in 2000 while denying risk. Washington, D.C. *Health Letter*, Public Citizen's Health Research Group, August 2005: 1-2.

18. Larkin, M. Whose article is it anyway? *Lancet* 353: 136, 1999.

19. Lexchin, J, Bero, LA, Djulbegovic, B et al. Pharmaceutical industry sponsorship and research outcome and quality: A systematic review. *BMJ* 326: 1167, 2003.

20. Erichacker, PQ, Natanson, C, Danner, RL. Surviving sepsis—practice guidelines, marketing campaigns, and Eli Lilli. *N Engl J Med* 355 (16): 1640-1642, 2006.

21. Abboud, L, Zuckerman, G. Drug maker draws heat for sharing non-public data with stock analysts. *Wall Street Journal*, October 4, 2005.

22. Krumhholtz, SD, Egilman, DS, Ross, JS. Study of Neurontin: titrate to effect, profile of safety (STEPS) trial. *Arch Intern Med* 171 (12):1100-1107, 2011.

23. Feigal, DW, Gardner, SN, McClellan, J. Ensuring safe and effective medical devices. *N Engl J Med* 348: 191, 2003.

24. Burton, TM, Mathews, AW. Guidant sold heart device after flaws. *Wall Street Journal*, June 2, 2005: D3.

25. Meier, B. Hip implants U.S. rejected sold overseas. *New York Times*, February 12, 2012: A1.

26. Higginson, G. Political considerations for changing medical screening programs. *JAMA* 282: 1472-1474, 1999.

27. Ubel, PA, Asch, DA. Creating value in health by understanding and overcoming resistance to de-innovation. *Health Affairs* 34 (2): 239-244, 2015.

28. Perry, S. The brief life of the National Center for Health Care Technology. *N Engl J Med* 307: 1095-1100, 1982.

29. Mervis, J. Technology assessment faces ax. *Science* 266: 1636, 1994.

30. Leary, WE. Congress's science agency prepares to close its doors. *New York Times,* September 24, 1995: A26.

31. Holtz, RL. What you didn't know about a drug can hurt you: Untold numbers of clinical trial results go unpublished; those that are made public can't always be believed. *Wall Street Journal,* December 12, 2008: A16.

32. Wang, SS. FDA panel takes a second look. *Wall Street Journal,* September 8, 2011: B6.

33. Abelson, R, Pollack, A. Medicare widens drugs it accepts for cancer care: More off-label uses. *New York Times,* January 27, 2009.

34. Saluja, S, Woolhandler, S, Himmelstein, DU et al. *Intl J Health Services,* June 14, 2016.

35. Demko, P. Healthcare's hired hands: When the stakes rise in Washington, healthcare interests seek well-connected lobbying firms. *Modern Healthcare,* October 6, 2014.

36. Brenner, DJ, Hall, EJ. Computed tomography—an increasing source of radiation exposure. *N Engl J Med* 357: 2277-2284, 2007.

37. Helliker, K. The case for fewer fetal scans. *Wall Street Journal,* July 18-19, 2016: A1.

CHAPTER 4

INCREASING SPECIALIZATION AND
SUB-SPECIALIZATION

One of the most dramatic changes in U.S. medicine over these last 60 years has been the exponential growth in specialization and sub-specialization. Here we will look at this trend and its implications for the future.

Some Historical Perspective

The tension between generalists and specialists goes back much farther in history than we might expect. Before 2000 BC, Herodotus described medical practice in the Nile valley of Egypt this way:

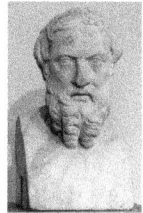

> *The art of medicine is thus divided: each physician applies himself to one disease only and not more. All places abound in physicians; some are for the eyes, others for the head, others for the teeth, others for the intestines, and others for internal disorders.* [1]

Will Rogers (1879-1935) saw the matter this way:

> *This is a day of specializing, especially with the doctors. Say, for instance, there is something the matter with your right eye. You go to a doctor, and he tells you, 'I'm sorry, but I am a left-eye doctor; I make a specialty of left eyes.' Take the throat business, for instance. A doctor that doctors on the upper part of the throat, he*

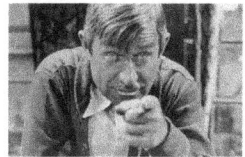

doesn't know where the lower part goes to. And the highest priced one of all of them is another bird that just tells you which doctor to go to. He can't cure even corns or open a boil himself. He is a Diagnostician, but he's nothing but a traffic cop, to direct ailing people.

The old-fashioned doctor didn't pick out a big toe or left ear to make a life's living on. He picked the whole human frame. No matter what end of you was wrong, he had to try to cure you single handed.

In 1900, when more that 80 percent of American physicians were in general practice, this editorial appeared in *The Journal of the American Medical Association*:

In these days of specialization, the field of the general practitioner is becoming greatly restricted. In fact, there is some danger that in many instances the so-called general practitioner ultimately may come to perform the functions of a mere business agent of the specialists, and to act as the local distributor for the patients in his community. At the same time, as the value and the need of genuine specialists in medicine are fully recognized and established, there cannot be too strong a warning uttered against a tendency noticeable in some quarters to carry specialization to a degree of refinement beyond all reason. [2]

Table 4.1 shows the years that specialty boards were established in this country up until 1980. Some of the specialty boards were defined by anatomy (e.g. ophthalmology and dermatology), one by gender (obstetrics-gynecology) two by age (pediatrics and internal medicine), and many by basic approach to treatment (most surgical specialties).

In 1970, Wayne G. Menke, Ph.D. of the National Academy of Sciences noted the dilemma being created by specialization in these words:

Specialization is both a product of and a contributor to the scientific information explosion in medicine. It subdivides both doctor and patient, increases the difficulty of attaining a clear sense of medical identity for students and young physicians, and places additional strain on the traditional doctor-patient relationship. Specialization emphasizes the science of medicine and its rational processes in the treatment of disease and contributes to depersonalization, aggravates patient anxieties, and implicitly encourages quackery. It is probably the major factor disturbing traditional ethical and economic patterns in medicine, and it dominates medical education and research and medical practice, promotes jurisdictional disputes within the profession, and weakens organizational strength and professional power. [3]

TABLE 4.1

YEARS OF ORGANIZATION OF SPECIALTY BOARDS

Board	Year	Board	Year
Ophthalmology	1917	Surgery	1937
Otolaryngology	1924	Anesthesiology	1938
Obstetrics-gynecology	1930	Plastic surgery	1939
Dermatology	1932	Neurologic surgery	1940
Pediatrics	1933	Physical medicine and rehabilitation	1947
Orthopedic surgery	1934	Preventive medicine	1948
Psychiatry-neurology	1934	Thoracic surgery	1950
Radiology	1934	Family practice	1969
Colon-rectal surgery	1935	Allergy and immunology	1971
Urology	1935	Nuclear medicine	1971
Internal medicine	1936	Emergency medicine	1979
Pathology	1936	Medical genetics	1991

Source: Geyman, JP. *Health Care in America: Can Our Ailing System be Healed?* Boston. *Butterworth Heinemann*, 2002, p.45

The trend toward increasing specialization was accelerated after World War II. General practice had no significant place in our medical schools, and medical students had little or no contact with general practitioners. General practice was declining without the academic, educational and research components that it needed as its own clinical discipline. Many generalists, often in solo practice, became overburdened in uncontrolled practices and left to train in a more limited specialty residency.

By the 1960s, there was a growing concern that generalist physicians were being replaced by too many specialists, raising questions over whether our physician workforce had the best balance between generalists and specialists to meet the needs of our population for health care. A landmark study was published in 1961 by Dr. Kerr White and his colleagues at the University of North Carolina School of Medicine, "The Ecology of Medical Care." Based on studies in this country and in the U.K., they found that, in an average month, 750 adults out of a 1,000 will have an episode of illness; of these 237 will see a physician, but only 9 will be hospitalized, 5 will be referred to another physician, and 1 will be referred to a university medical center. Figure 4.1 shows these striking differences.

The authors of that study brought forward the importance of studying how, and how effectively, medical care is actually delivered, with this observation: [4]

> *Medical-care research is concerned with the problems of assessing needs and of delivering medical care; more specifically, it is concerned with problems of implementing the advances achieved by medical science. Its concerns are not the characteristics, prevalence and mechanisms of disease, but the social, psychologic, cultural, economic,*

*informational, administrative, and organizational factors
that inhibit and facilitate access to and delivery of the best
contemporary health care to individuals and communities.*

FIGURE 4.1

THE ECOLOGY OF MEDICAL CARE

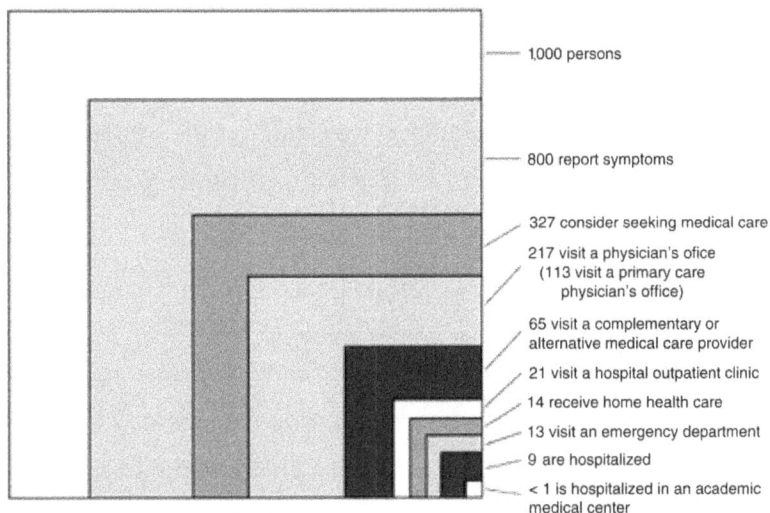

1,000 persons

800 report symptoms

327 consider seeking medical care

217 visit a physician's ofice
(113 visit a primary care
physician's office)

65 visit a complementary or
alternative medical care provider

21 visit a hospital outpatient clinic

14 receive home health care

13 visit an emergency department

9 are hospitalized

< 1 is hospitalized in an academic
medical center

Source: White, KL, Williams, TF, Greenberg, BG. The Ecology of Medical Care. *N Engl J Med* 265:885-892, 1961. Reprinted with permission.

Not only did research on medical care itself take on new importance in the 1960s, but American medicine became a bit more introspective in recognizing its shortcomings. Four major studies were carried out by independent groups in the mid-1960s, all of which came to the same conclusion—more generalist physicians needed to be trained to serve as the foundation of our health care system. [5-8] These reports led to the creation of family practice as the nation's 20th specialty in 1969. At that time, Dr. Richard Magraw captured the essence of this re-direction in his book, *Ferment in Medicine* in these words:

> *Specialization thus pervades American medicine to-*
> *day and shows every sign of increasing. Yet an individual*
> *(meaning literally indivisible or not dividable) is a whole,*
> *standing in persistent and perverse opposition to the focus*
> *of the specialty, which is by definition a fragment. . . . We*
> *make an important mistake in emphasis when we talk of*
> *problems of specialization in medicine. Our real problems*
> *are those of coordination and integration.* [9]

In the 1970s, more attention was paid to the generalist base of medicine as the five essential attributes of primary medical care were defined—*accessibility, comprehensiveness, coordination, continuity, and accountability.* [10] Primary care physicians were on the front lines of medical practice, were able to manage most common problems that patients brought to them, and were starting to evolve group practices. They were becoming more recognized in medical schools and teaching hospitals in three kinds of programs: family practice, general internal medicine, and general pediatrics.

But despite this progress, the balance between generalists and non-primary care specialties continued to shift away from the nation's need for primary care as the foundation of our system. The proportions of generalists among the national physician workforce declined from 43 percent in 1965 to less than 30 percent in 1990, when only 11.5 percent were in general/family practice. (Figure 4.2)[11]

Continued specialization and sub-specialization has continued unabated in recent decades as a growing maldistribution by specialty has become the norm. The American Board of Medical Specialties today has some 150 member boards and certified sub-specialties.

Less than 20 percent of physicians today are in primary care as the nation faces a shortage of 52,000 primary care physicians

FIGURE 4.2

PERCENTAGE OF TOTAL PHYSICIANS: PRIMARY CARE SPECIALTIES

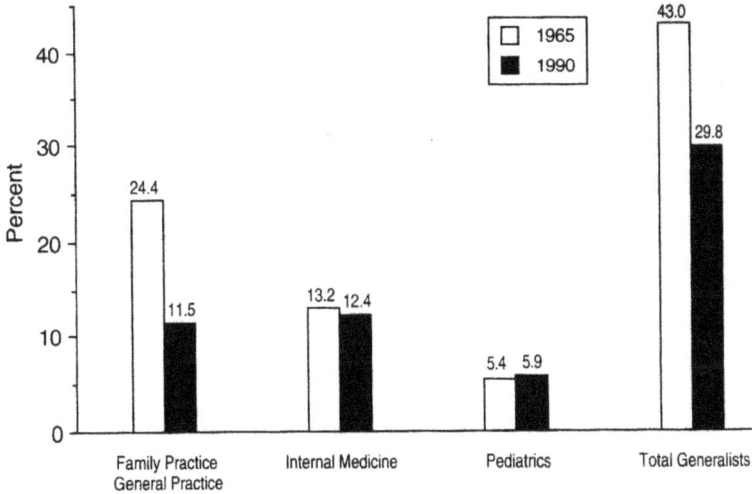

Source: Schroeder, SA The Troubled Profession: Is medicine's glass half-full or half-empty? *Ann Intern Med* 116: 583-592, 1992. Reprinted with permission.

by 2025. [12] Family medicine, as the direct descendent of general practice, taking care of patients regardless of age, comprises less than 10 percent of the country's physician workforce, despite having established itself in medical schools and teaching hospitals. The large majority of internists and pediatricians enter one or another subspecialty. The growing specialty maldistribution of physicians is due in large part to the higher reimbursement of procedural and non-primary care services. That has led to shortages in the more time-intensive specialties, also including geriatrics and psychiatry.

Impacts of Specialty Maldistribution on Patient Care

Primary care by definition includes *all* of these four basic features: (1) first-contact care; (2) longitudinal continuity of care over time; (3) comprehensiveness, with capacity to manage the majority of health problems that patients present with; and (4) coordination of care with other parts of the health care system. [13] Some specialties can deal with some of these services, such as emergency medicine physicians for first-contact care or opthalmologists providing continuity of eye care over years, but are not doing primary care.

As a result of the primary care shortage, patients with acute problems often have a hard time seeing a physician. In 2010, only 42 percent of 353 million annual visits for acute care in the U.S. were made to patients' personal physicians; 28 percent were seen in emergency rooms (with no continuity of subsequent care), 20 percent to non-primary care specialists, and 7 percent to hospital outpatient departments, again with difficulty in arranging follow-up. [14] Patients with different kinds of chronic health problems often need to see several other specialists for their ongoing care, each without a comprehensive range of skills, who often prescribe medications that conflict with patients' other medications.

In past years, primary care physicians would care for their patients in the hospital when hospitalization was required, which was good in terms of continuity of care and knowledge of what the patient and his or her family wanted and needed. That continuity is largely gone today as hospitalists have become the norm to oversee care in the hospital. They have not seen the patient before, have little awareness of the patient's other health problems or circumstances, and tend to "ping pong" the patient to other specialists in the hospital, often again who have not previously seen the patient.

As a result of decreasing continuity of care, patients incur increased costs, less coordination, decreased quality of care, and often worse outcomes. Past studies have documented that areas of the country with more primary care physicians have less use of intensive services, lower costs, and higher quality of care. [15] By contrast, patients in areas with a surplus of non-primary care specialists are

more likely to have late-stage colorectal cancer when first diagnosed, as well as worse outcomes. [16]

Although there have been various efforts at the national level
in recent decades to develop a physician workforce plan that best
meets the needs of our population for ready access to primary care,
the above shows that we still do not have such a plan. We will consider some of the reasons for this failure in the next chapter, and
what the implications are for our health care system.

Endnotes:

1. Margotta, R. *The Story of Medicine*. New York. *Golden Press*, 1968, p. 25.
2. Editorial. *JAMA* 232: 1420, 1900.
3. Menke, WG. Divided labor: the doctor as specialist. *Ann Intern Med* 72: 943, 1970.
4. White, KL, Williams, F, Greenberg, BG. The ecology of medical care. *N Engl J Med* 265:885-892, 1961.
5. The graduate education of physicians. *The report of the Citizens Commission of Graduate Medical Education*, Chicago, AMA, 1966.
6. Meeting the challenge of family practice. *The report of the Ad Hoc Committee on Education for Family Practice of the Council on Medical Education*, Chicago, AMA, 1966.
7. Health is a community affair. *The report of the National Commission on Community Health Services*. Pub. *Harvard University Press*, Cambridge, MA, 1966.
8. Editorial. The core content of family medicine, report of the committee on requirements for certification. *GP* 34: 225, 1966.
9. Magraw, RM. *Ferment in Medicine*. Philadelphia, *W. B. Saunders Company*, 1966, p. 154.
10. A manpower policy for primary health care. Washington, D.C.: *Institute of Medicine, National Academy of Sciences,* 16-26, 1978.
11. Schroeder, SA. The troubled profession: is medicine's glass half full or half empty? *Ann Intern Med* 116: 583-592, 1992.
12. Peterson, SM, Liaw, WR, Phillips, RL et al. Projecting U.S. primary care physician workforce needs: 2010-2025. *Ann Fam Med* 10 (6): 503-509, 2012.
13. Starfield, B. Is primary care essential? *The Lancet* 344 (8930): 1129-1133, 1994.

14. Pitts, SR, Carrier, ER, Rich, EC et al. Where Americans get acute care: increasingly, it's not at their doctor's office. *Health Affairs* 29 (5): 1620-1628, 2010.

15. Parchman, M, Culter, S. Primary care physicians and avoidable hospitalizations. *J Fam Pract* 39: 123-126, 1994.

16. Roetzheim, RG, Pal, N, Gonzalez, EC et al. The effects of physician supply on the early detection of colorectal cancer. *J Fam Pract* 48 (11): 850-858, 1999.

CHAPTER 5

DECLINE AND FRAGMENTATION
OF PRIMARY CARE

As we saw in the last chapter, primary care has been going downhill in this country for a long time, despite incremental attempts since the 1970s to reverse the process. We noted the five criteria for primary care services—*accessibility, comprehensiveness, coordination, continuity, and accountability*—as the purview and responsibility of primary care physicians. In 1975, Dr. Gayle Stephens, long-time family physician, educator and scholar, summed up this essential role in these words:

> *The sine qua non is the knowledge and skill that allows a physician to confront relatively large numbers of unselected patients with unselected conditions and to carry on therapeutic relationships with patients.* [1]

That's what all of us general practitioners were trained to do, and did effectively, 60 years ago. And, as we saw in the last chapter, that is what is largely absent today, despite efforts to rebuild primary care as the foundation of our health care system.

What's Been Done about Specialty Mal-Distribution?

With the emerging concern in the late 1960s that the generalist base of our system needed to be rebuilt, incremental steps were taken in that direction, including establishing family medicine, general internal medicine, and general pediatrics programs in most medical schools, increasing their funding, and various efforts to foster their collaboration. Some successes were achieved, but these three disciplines often competed, such as for space and resources, more than collaborated with each other. Meanwhile, medical students were finding that specialists still dominated academic medical centers and most of their other educational settings, and that many had little regard for or understanding of primary care.

In 1972, the Coordinating Council on Medical Education (CCME) was established under the umbrella of five parent organizations: the American Board of Medical Specialties, the American Hospital Association, the American Medical Association, the Association of American Medical Colleges, and the Council on Medical Specialty Societies. This group was charged with the responsibility to analyze the nation's problem with specialty distribution and to recommend remedial approaches to meet national requirements for health care. But the CCME declined to accept any regulatory function, offered at one point under a contract with the federal Department of Health, Education and Welfare, and was ineffective in its task. [2]

In 1992, the Council on Graduate Medical Education (COGME) issued an important report, *Improving Access to Health Care through Physician Workforce Reform: Directions for the 21st Century*, setting a long-term national goal of 50 percent of residency graduates practicing in one of the three primary care specialties. These are some of their recommendations:

1. *Establishing a national physician commission and state physician commissions.*
2. *Implementing the manpower plan through consortia that might include medical schools, teaching hospitals, community health centers, health maintenance organizations, and other educational entities.*

3. *Allocating graduate medical education positions and funding based on local and regional needs, and*

4. *Providing increased incentives for primary care practice in underserved, inner city, and rural areas.* [3]

Logical and needed as these recommendations were, however, this planning never resulted in real system change. To be sure, some institutions, such as the University of Washington's WAMI program, the University of Minnesota's Duluth program, and Thomas Jefferson University's Physician Shortage Area Program, have made major strides in training more primary care physicians to better serve their regional needs for physicians. But there was no central responsibility for the specialty mix of residency positions at the national or state level. Teaching hospitals could continue to unilaterally increase their own residency and fellowship positions in non-primary care disciplines in response to their own service or financial needs without regard to regional or national needs, and still be reimbursed for such increases by the Health Care Financing Administration in a policy-neutral way.

In 2001, Gayle Stephens had this to say about paralysis of meaningful change:

> *Among the lessons that ought to have been learned during the last 30 years is that the 'natural' evolution of change is not necessarily in the public interest; that the bête noir of change is not 'socialized medicine' as the AMA tirelessly warned us for decades—compared to the draconian intrusions of industrialized medicine on free choice and privacy; and that organized medicine, hospitals, and medical schools are not dependable fountains of wisdom and leadership in the midst of change. Our 'expert' institutions and organizations have exposed themselves to be*

bastions of self-interest, and exploiters of the public purse. More than anything else, they resemble the medieval clergy in maintaining their death-grip on privilege, power, and self-aggrandizement. [4]

We are left today with this paradox—we are at a time that requires many more primary care physicians (the demand has never been greater), but we still have no consensus about a national physician workforce plan and continue with an inadequate capacity to re-balance the mix between generalist primary care physicians and the non-primary care specialties. Federal Title VII funds supporting primary care training programs were sharply reduced between 1977 and 2009. [5] Over the last 50 years, the medical education system has changed only at the margins while the practice environment, through our reimbursement policies, continues to favor non-primary care specialists over primary care. Graduating medical students are heavily burdened with debt often between $150,000 and $200,000. As they look at projected gaps in career incomes between specialists and primary care (Figure 5.1) [6], they naturally see the advantages of the better reimbursed non-primary care fields. It is no surprise, then, to find the ROAD specialties (radiology, orthopedic surgery, anesthesiology, and dermatology) are most attractive to medical school graduates.

Increasing Fragmentation of Primary Care

Even as the shortage of primary care physicians grows, primary care itself is becoming increasingly fragmented. A landmark 2002 article, *Family Practice in the United States: position and prospects*, gave us a snapshot of the primary care landscape in the early 2000s, showing a rapidly changing environment so different from the central role played by generalist physicians 60 years ago. Here are examples of these changes at the start of this century: [7]

FIGURE 5.1

Annual Ordinary Income, Before Taxe For Various Professional and Educational Attainment Levels, Ages 22-65

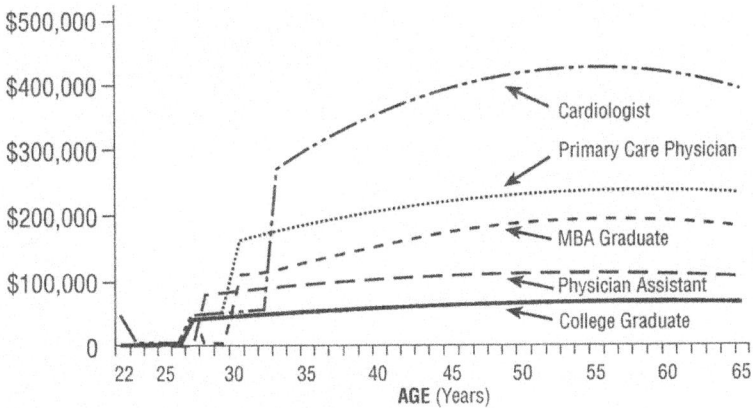

Source: Reprinted with permission from Vaughn, BT, DeVrieze, SR, Reed, SD, Schullman, JA. Can we close the income gap between specialists and primary care physicians? *Health Affairs* 29 (5): 933-40, 2010.

- In aggregate, the proportion of family physicians and general practitioners (then only about 10 percent of the U.S. physician workforce), had declined since 1970.

- Internal medicine and pediatrics were expected to see another surge in sub-specialization. [8]

- By 2000, there were more nurse practitioners in the U.S. (about 102,000) than general practice/family medicine combined, with about 90 percent working in primary care and licensed in many states to practice independently from physicians; in addition, there were about 45,000 physician assistants, with about one-half of them working with primary care physicians. [9]

- Alternative care providers were estimated to account for more visits each year in the U.S. than visits to all primary care physicians, with out-of-pocket costs exceeding those for all U.S. hospitalizations. [10]

- Psychologists were authorized in New Mexico to prescribe psychotropic drugs. [11]

- Medicaid was reimbursing chiropractic in 33 states, biofeedback in 10 states, acupuncture in 7 states, hypnotherapy in 5 states, and massage therapy in 2 states. [12]

- Naturopaths were licensed in 12 states, and insurance companies in Washington and Connecticut were required to cover their services. [13]

- "Pharmaceutical care" by pharmacists was a steadily growing trend, with more than 30 states allowing some form of collaborative management with physicians for selection, initiation, monitoring, or modifying a patient's drug therapy, as well as allowing them to give immunizations independently in 30 states.[14]

- Self-care by patients was taking many new forms, such as through diagnostic and screening tests, even including patients getting full-body CT scans without their physician's involvement [15], as well as drugs marketed directly to the public, and patients being able to directly purchase drugs without their physician's prescription through rapidly growing mail-order pharmacies and Internet sources. [16]

The growing numbers of nurse practitioners and physician assistants, together with an increasing emphasis on team practice, has led to improvement of primary care in many settings. But this advance has seen limits as well. More than one-half of nurse practitioners and physician assistants are practicing in non-primary care specialties and sub-specialties, ranging from orthopedic surgery to renal dialysis and infertility. Again, predictably, many are attracted by the same things that attract so many physicians—the higher salaries in specialists' practices. [17]

In his excellent 2010 book, *Practice Under Pressure: Primary Care Physicians and Their Medicine in the Twenty-First Century*, Timothy Hoff, associate professor of health policy and management at the University of Albany School of Public Health, described the dysfunctional business model for U.S. primary care in this way:

> *The halcyon days of generalist care, where primary care physicians (PCPs) alone determined the scope, substance, and economic value of all primary care work have been replaced by an environment in which PCPs must make serious choices about which work to keep, which to jettison, and how to maintain job and patient satisfaction within a rigidly imposed reimbursement model that favors quick episodic care. The twenty-first century U.S. health care system now pays PCPs less for the same type of care, ignores the practice of cognitive medicine that involves skills such as history taking and counseling, demands that PCPs see lots of patients in a given day to break even, motivates PCPs to give up low-margin parts of their business regardless of the personal or patient-related benefits derived from having PCPs engaged in that business . . . Where the generalist of 1970 could spend forty-five minutes talking with a patient and be paid for that time, now insurers affix precise dollar amounts and time limits to different clinical diagnoses. This leaves PCPs little discretion to make their own judgments about whether or not more time is needed with a particular patient.* [18]

Other trends in more recent years have further eroded the whole concept of a primary care physician working at the foundation of primary care. These include the rapid growth of urgent care clinics and emergency facilities affiliated with hospitals, and retail clinics in shopping malls, chain drug stores and other big retailers. These clinics are typically staffed by nurse practitioners for "convenience care." While these kinds of facilities can provide access to first-contact care, note that they lack follow-up care as well as the four other requirements of primary care—comprehensiveness, coordination, continuity, and accountability. Continuity and coordination of care are further limited by after-hours call arrangements within larger group practices, withdrawal of primary care physicians from hospital care, increasing mobility of both patients and physicians, and growing instability of health plan coverage that often results in patients having to change physicians. Solo and small-group family practices, which used to be the cornerstone of continuity of care, are disappearing with more than 60 percent of U.S. physicians now employed by large hospital systems.

Implications of Specialty Mal-Distribution on Our Health Care System

We have seen that unfettered markets fuel specialization and sub-specialization in the medical education environment as well as in the clinical practice environment. Free markets end up producing more physician specialists in the non-primary care fields, especially given the lack of a national or state physician manpower plan that would best meet society's needs for primary care. We have also seen that modest gains in medical education have failed to alter the structure, values, and mission of academic medical centers while leaving in place all the disincentives to generalist practice in the practice environment.

Why does all this matter? As other advanced nations learned long ago, it is only logical and rational to base their health care systems on a primary care base, in line with the classic "ecology of medical care" mentioned earlier. At the base of the system is a primary care foundation, readily accessible to patients with unselected and common health care problems. Secondary care involves more specialized care, available on referral to nearby specialists and sub-specialists, with tertiary care provided for unusual or rare medical problems by sub-specialists in academic medical centers. (Figure 5.2) [19] In this kind of system, the main differences between primary care physicians and consulting referral physicians are summarized in Table 5.1. [20]

FIGURE 5.2

Levels of Health Care

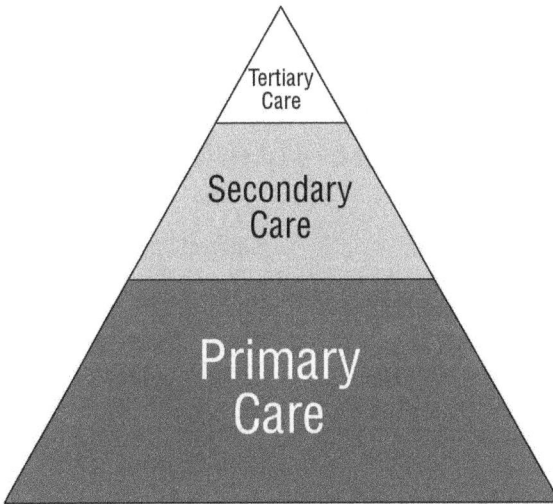

Source: Geyman, JP. *Breaking Point: How the Primary Care Crisis Endangers the Lives of Americans*, Friday Harbor, WA *Copernicus Healthcare* 2011 p. 47.

In its 2008 report, *Primary Health Care: Now More than Ever*, the World Health Organization updated its 1978 Declaration on Primary Care with this statement:

Essential features of a strong health system led by primary care are: accessibility (with no out-of-pocket payments), a person (not a disease) focus over time, universality, a broad range of services in primary care, and coordination when people do have to receive care elsewhere. . . Evidence at the macro level (e.g. policy, payment, regulations) is now overwhelming: countries with a strong service for primary care have better health outcomes at low cost. Systems that explicitly distribute resources according to population health needs (rather than demands), that eliminate co-payments, that assume responsibility for the financing of services within the primary care sector are more cost effective. [21]

TABLE 5.1

Characteristics of Physicians that May Affect Decision-Making Style

Primary Care Physician	Referral Physician
• Deals with multiple problems and diffuse complaints	• Asked to focus on one problem
• Longitudinal partnerships	• Brief relationship
• Knows the patient's character	• Relative stranger
• Knows the psychological setting of illness	• Asked to solve the problem
• Knows pattern of health complaints	• Intermediate to high probabilities of disease
• Can tolerate uncertainty	
• All probabilities of disease	

Source: Sox HC. Decision-making: A comparison of referral practice and primary care. *J Fam Pract.* 1996;42:156.

Instead of that logic, the U.S. has an inverted pyramid,with a small primary care sector atop that upside-down pyramid. As a result, the U.S. compares poorly with other advanced countries in terms of access, costs, and outcomes of care. The latest survey by the Commonwealth Fund compared 13 advanced countries and again, as in earlier surveys, the other countries fare much better. Figure 5.3 compares health care spending as a percentage of GDP in these countries from 1980 to 2013. High health care spending appears to be driven by greater use of medical technology and higher prices, rather than more physician visits or hospitalizations. Despite our spending so much, Americans have less access and worse outcomes of care, including the lowest life expectancy and the highest infant mortality rate among the countries studied, as well as a higher prevalence of chronic diseases. (Figure 5.3) [22]

FIGURE 5.3

HEALTH CARE SPENDING AS A PERCENTAGE OF GDP 1980-2013

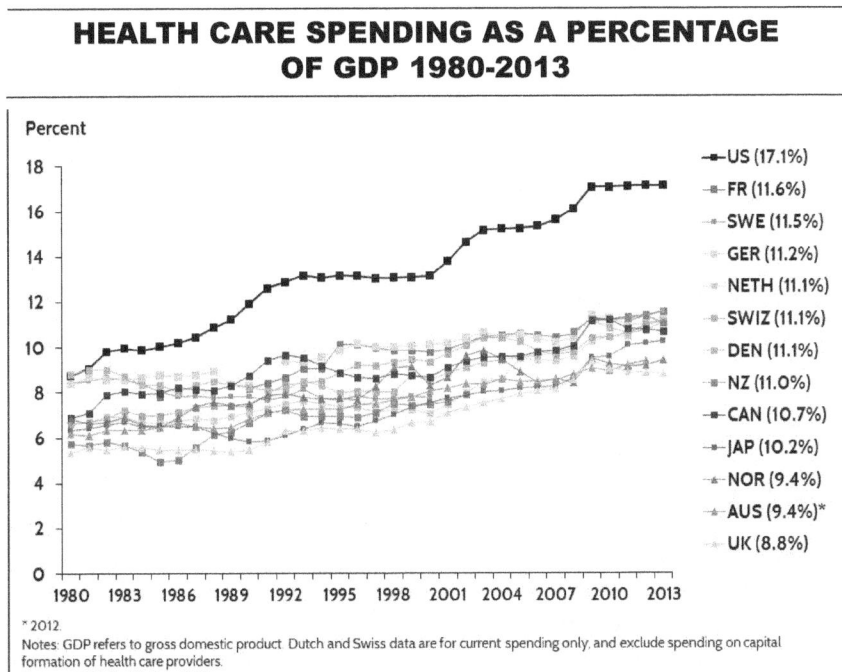

Notes: GDP refers to gross domestic product. Dutch and Swiss data are for current spending only, and exclude spending on capital formation of health care providers.

Source: OECD Health Data 2015

Unfortunately, the corporate stakeholders in the minimally-regulated marketplace of our medical-industrial complex do just fine with this situation at the expense of patients, families and taxpayers. Our so-called health care system is unsustainable on its present course without fundamental reform, which we will discuss in Part Three of this book. Meanwhile, it is time to move to the next chapter to consider a major culprit of our dysfunctional health care system—the soaring prices and costs of health care, with no containment in sight.

Endnotes:

1. Stephens, GG. The intellectual basis of family practice. *J Fam Pract* 2 (4): 428, 1975.
2. Specialty distribution and the CCME. *J Med Educ* 52: 861-862, 1977.
3. Council on Graduate Medical Education. Third report. *Improving Access to Health Care through Physician Workforce Reform: Directions for the 21st Century.* Rockville, MD: U.S. Department of Health and Human Services, Public Health Service Health Resources and Services Administration, Bureau of Health Professions, Division of Medicine, 11, 12, 48, 68-70, 1992.
4. Stephens, GG. Family practice and social and political change. In Keystone III: the role of family practice in a changing health care environment: a dialogue. Washington, D.C. Robert Graham Center, 230-233, 2001.
5. Robert Graham Center. *Title VII's decline: shrinking investment in the primary care training pipeline.* Washington, D.C. The Robert Graham Center for Policy Studies in Family Medicine and Primary Care, 2009.
6. Vaughn, BT, DeVrieze, SR, Reed, SD et al. Can we close the income gap between specialists and primary care physicians? *Health Affairs* 29 (5): 933-940, 2010.
7. Green, LA, Fryer, GE. Family practice in the United States: position and prospects. *Acad Med* 77: 787-789, 2002.
8. Terry, K. What's on the horizon for primary care? *Med Econ* 8: 27-31, 2002.
9. Hooker, RS, McCaig, LF. Use of physician assistants and nurse practitioners in primary care, 1995-1999. Health Aff (Millwood) 20 (4): 231-238, 2001.
10. Eisenberg, DM, Davis, RB, Ettner, SL et al. Trends in alternative medicine use in the United States, 1990-1997: results of a follow-up national survey. *JAMA* 280: 1569-1575, 1998.
11. Gloor, J. New Mexico psychologists gain prescribing privileges. *Family Practice Report* 8 (4): 1, 2002.
12. Brunk, D. Some alternative treatments covered by Medicaid plans. *Family Practice News* 1: 44, 2000.

13. Peterson, A. States grant "herb doctors" new powers. *Wall Street Journal,* August 22, 2002: D1.

14. Pharmacists finding solutions through collaboration, volume 2002. Alliance for Pharmaceutical Care, Partners to Improve Health Outcomes. www.accp.com/position/paper10.pdf. Accessed February 1, 2001.

15. Lee, TH, Brennan, TA. Direct-to-consumer marketing of high-technology screening tests. *N Engl J Med* 346: 529, 2003.

16. Practice trends. Cheap drugs for American seniors. *Family Practice News* 33 (8): 42, 2003.

17. Rollet, J. 2009 Nurse Salary & Workplace Survey: good news in troubled economy. *Adv Nurse Pract* 18 (1): 24-26, 29-30, 2010.

18. Hoff, T. *Practice Under Pressure: Primary Care Physicians and Their Medicine in the Twenty-First Century.* Piscataway, NJ. *Rutgers University Press*, 2010, pp. 16-17.

19. Geyman, JP. *Breaking Point: How the Primary Care Crisis Endangers the Lives of Americans.* Friday Harbor, WA. *Copernicus Healthcare*, 2011, p. 47.

20. Sox, HC. Decision-making: A comparison of referral practice and primary care. *J Fam Pract* 42: 156, 1996.

21. Rawaf, S, De Maeseneer, J, Starfield, B. From Alma-Ata to Almaty: A new start for primary health care. *The Lancet on line* 372, October 18, 2008.

22. Issue Brief. U.S. Health Care from a Global Perspective. Spending, use of services, prices, and health in 13 countries. *The Commonwealth Fund*, October 8, 2015.

CHAPTER 6

SOARING COSTS AND
UNAFFORDABILITY OF CARE

I find little evidence anywhere that market forces, bluntly used, that is, consumer choice among an array of products with competitors fighting it out, leads to a health care system you want and need. In the U.S. competition has become toxic: it is a major reason for our duplicative, supply-driven, fragmented health care system . . . Unfettered growth and pursuit of institutional self-interest has been the engine of low-value for the U.S. health care system. It has made it unaffordable, and hasn't helped patients at all. [1]

—Don Berwick, M.D., founder of the Institute for
Healthcare Improvement and former administrator of the
Centers for Medicare and Medicaid Services (CMS)

The threat of sky rocketing costs of health care in this country, without any cost containment in sight, poses a growing barrier to health care to much of our population and threatens patients and system alike with future bankruptcy. It results from many of the entrenched trends we've discussed in earlier chapters, including increasing specialization, declining primary care, increasing technology, corporatization, and increasing privatization with deregulated markets. It is one of the most striking changes in U.S. medicine over the last 60 years.

This chapter has three goals: (1) to review the long trends in inflating health care costs, together with how various industries have gamed the system in their own self-interest; (2) to consider the extent and impacts of the unaffordability of health care for ordinary Americans; and (3) to summarize some of the ineffective approaches that have been taken to rein in costs.

The Relentless Upward Climb of Health Care Costs

When I started practice in the early 1960s, health care costs comprised little more than 5 percent of GDP. As a curious piece of history, Table 6.1 shows the minimal fee schedule that was used in the Siskiyou County Medical Society in California in 1950 [2]; fees were slightly higher when I was in practice in Mount Shasta in the early 1960s.

Since then, health care costs have grown to almost 18 percent of GDP and are headed for 19.6 percent by 2024. [3] Figure 6.1 shows this ascent, compared to Canada, which effectively controlled health care costs after its single-payer financing plan was enacted in the early 1970s. Within total health care expenditures, almost one-third of the money goes to hospitals, nearly one-fifth to physician services, and slightly less than one-tenth to prescription drugs. [4]

It is interesting to calculate the differences in cost of living between 1960 and 2016. Annual inflation over this period was about 3.79 percent, representing about an eight-fold increase in the cost of living. [5] But health care costs today are much higher than this eight-fold increase.

Intended as it was to contain costs and make health care more affordable, has the ACA made a dent in this problem over the last six years? Figure 6.2 show how the answer is an unequivocal "No." In fact, U.S. national health care spending reached a new peak of $10,345 per person in 2016. [6]

TABLE 6.1

MINIMUM FEE SCHEDULE

Siskiyou County Medical Society

EFFECTIVE MAY 1, 1948

Procedure or Service:	Minimum Fee:
PATIENT VISITS	
Office—first complete	$5.00
routine, follow-up	3.00
Hospital—first complete	5.00
follow-up	4.00
Home—first complete	5.00
follow-up	4.80
night (10 p.m. to 7 a.m.)	7.00
Consultation	10.00
Mileage charge (per mile) one way, out of town limits	1.00
PRE- AND POST-NATAL CARE	
Pregnancy (complete)	$100.00
Caesarian Section	200.00
Curettage	80.00
Circumcision—infant	10.00
all other ages	35.00
Removal Cervical Polyp	60.00
Perineorrhaphy	$150–200.00
Hysterectomy	200.00
(simple, supracervical)	
FRACTURES (Examples)	
Forearm or leg—one bone	$30.00
two bones	52.50
Femur or humerus	75.00
Clavical or scapula	37.50
Ribs	10.00
Complicating features, casts, splints and after care extra.	

Procedure or Service:	Minimum Fee:
GENERAL SURGICAL PROCEDURES	
Abdominal Laparotomies	$150–200.00
Cholecystectomy	200.00
Gastroenterostomy	250.00
Bowel resection	250.00
Thyroidectomy	200.00
Tonsillectomy—children	50.00
adults	75.00
Herniorraphy—single	150.00
double	200.00
Hemorrhoidectomy	100.00
Injection treatment, each	5.00
Hydrocele repair	75.00
Nephrectomy	250.00
Prostatectomy	$200–250.00
Vasectomy	50.00
Ligation, Saphenous vein	75.00
MISCELLANEOUS	
Assistance to major surgery	$25.00
Transfusion	25.00
Wassermann (or other blood test)	5.00
Penicillin (300,000 units)	7.50
Streptomycin—per gram	7.50
Aspiration (any joint or cavity including hydrocale)	10.00
Anesthesia—inhalation, spinal or intravenous, administered by M. D. for major surgery	25.00
for minor surgery	$5–10.00
(including tonsillectomy)	
Gonorrhea—complete treatment with penicillin	50.00

These are minimum fees for individual uncomplicated procedures bound on average costs and average time consumption by the physician and also bound on the patient's income up to $3,000.00 per year. Variations from this basis in relation to the above minimum fees are expected to be dealt with fairly at the discretion of the physician who may otherwise jeopardize his ethical standing in the Siskiyou County Medical Society.

Source: Geyman, JP. *Health Care in America: Can Our Ailing System be Healed?* Boston. *Butterworth Heinemann*, 2002, p.94

How could we expect any other trend, when we look at how various industries within the medical-industrial complex game our "system" for maximal profits? These examples make the point:

FIGURE 6.1

HEALTH COSTS AS PERCENTAGE OF GDP:
U.S. and Canada, 1960-2017

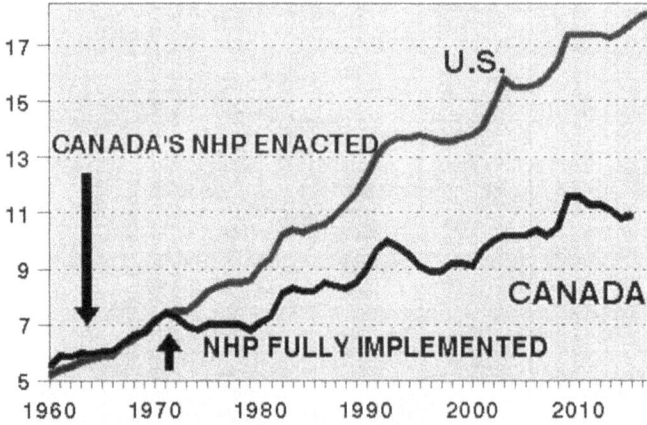

Source: Statistics Canada, Canadian Inst. for Health Info., & NCHS/Commerce Dept

FIGURE 6.2

2014 Growth Rates by Selected Sector, Before and After the Impact of the Affordable Care Act

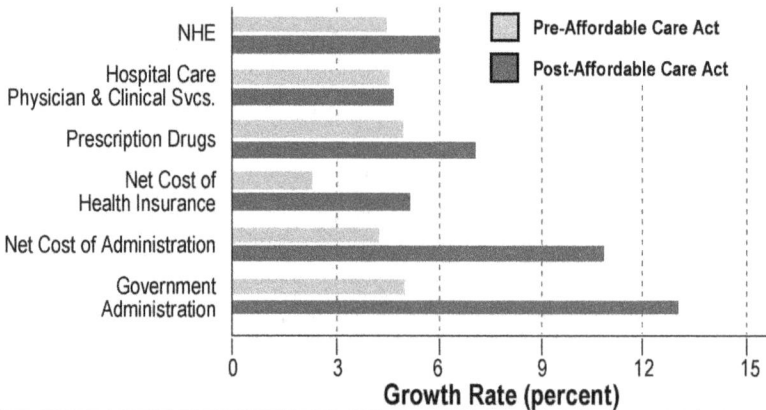

Source: Centers for Medicaid Services, Office of the Actuary, National Health Statistics Group, *Health Affairs*, October 2013.

Insurance industry

Insurers have all kinds of ways to increase their revenues by issuing policies with less and less value. These include high-deductible plans that won't even cover initial physicians' visits; changing, narrowed networks without out-of-network coverage; networks that exclude a majority of physicians and some major hospitals in an area; high co-insurance for specialty drugs; manipulation of risk scores to get higher Medicare payments; restrictive interpretations of what constitutes a medical emergency; marketing short-term plans lasting less that one year in order to avoid the ACA's coverage requirements; denial of services; exiting markets that aren't sufficiently profitable, and continued increases of premiums to what the market can bear. Leading insurers are seeking average premium increases of 20 percent for 2017, with some states much higher, such as 65 percent for individual health plans in Georgia. [7]

Hospital industry

As we saw in Chapter 1, expanding and consolidating hospital systems have wide latitude to set their own prices to what the market will bear. The costs of outpatient medical services go up sharply as hospitals buy up more medical groups. [8] The costs of cardiac imaging are two to three times higher when performed in hospital outpatient departments compared to physicians' offices. [9] There are also extreme variations in charges, especially among for-profit hospitals, for the same services e.g. charges in California for an uncomplicated Caesarian section ranging from $8,312 to $70,908. [10] (As you will see in Chapter 15, the cost for the physician's fee for a Caesarian section, including all prenatal and postpartum care, was about $300 in the early 1960s!) Hospitals also have many ways to game the reimbursement system, such as using "observation days" to count toward CMS's rules requiring three minimum inpatient days before follow-up nursing home care will be covered [11], and timing patient discharges from long-term hospitals to maximize Medicare reimbursement. [12] Administrative costs of U.S. hospitals are far higher than elsewhere around the world—25.3 percent of total hospital expenditures, compared to about 12 percent in Scotland and Canada, both of which have single-payer systems paying hospitals by global operating budgets. [13]

Drug industry

In part driven by intense direct-to-consumer drug advertising (DTCA) since the 1990s, the use of prescription drugs by Americans has reached an all-time high. Now that many drugs for common conditions are losing their patent protection, the industry is shifting to TV ads for new, very expensive specialty drugs for less common conditions, such as Opdivo for lung cancer ($12,500 a month) and Hetlioz for a sleep disorder ($148,000 a year). [14] Many people take five or more medications, especially older patients with one or more chronic conditions, typically prescribed by different specialists, with a high prevalence of drug interactions. The industry has successfully warded off price controls for many years, and prices its drugs to and beyond what the market will bear.

Big PhRMA lobbies hard to avoid any price controls, claiming that they would reduce innovation and that their costs of R & D are so high. These claims are false, since many new drugs are developed overseas and R&D costs are exaggerated. Instead, the drug industry enjoys a huge return on investment, as shown in Figure 6.3.

Generic drugs in the past were a protection against these price increases, but no longer are, with some drugs increased by up to 1,000 percent, especially when there is little competition due to consolidation or when manufacturing quality problems cause shortages.[15] As one example, hospitals and pharmacies found the prices they had to pay for a bottle of 500 tablets of Doxycyline, a decades-old antibiotic, rose in just six months in 2014 from $20 to $1,849! [16]

FIGURE 6.3

DRUG COMPANY PROFITS, 1995-2015

Return on Revenues (%)

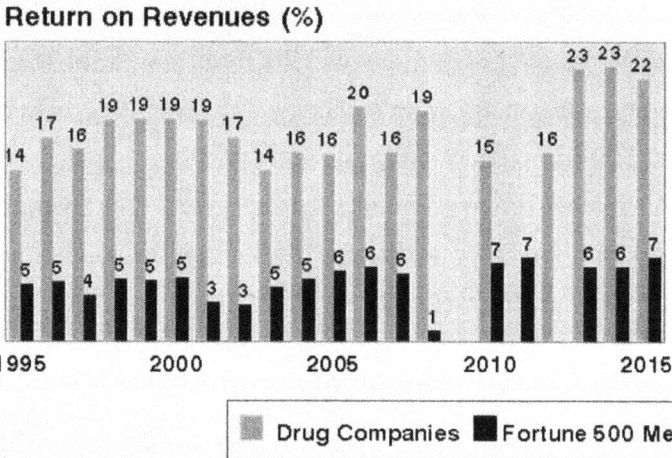

Source: Fortune 500 rankings for 1995-2016

Total drug company profits, 2015 = $67.1 billion

More than a half-million Americans were paying more than $50,000 for medications in 2014, up by 63 percent from 2013. [17]

Comparisons with other countries are staggering—in England and Norway, for example, Herceptin, a breast cancer drug, costs 30 and 28 percent, respectively, of what we pay here. [18] The Trans-Pacific Partnership Agreement (TPP), opposed by President Trump, would have driven up global drug prices further. [19]

In response to these soaring prices of drugs, both the AMA and the American Society of Health System Pharmacists have called for a ban on DTC ads. [20]

Physicians

As we will see in Chapter 13, physicians used to have a lot of autonomy in how they set up their practices. That is largely gone as almost two-thirds are employees of hospital systems or other large corporate group practices. They are under the thumb of system managers who expect them to be "productive" in maximizing revenue through shorter visits and higher volume, plus documenting the electronic record to facilitate up-coding for billing. Physicians often have little bargaining power in this new environment. As physicians consolidate in bigger groups in concentrated markets, their prices go up. [21] Stories abound of outrageous bills for minor problems, such as a tiny white spot on a patient's cheek soon generating bills of more than $25,000 from a dermatologist and anesthesiologist. [22] As insurers try to ratchet down payments to physicians and hospitals, they often react by charging additional fees, such as ophthalmologists charging separate "refraction fees" to measure visual acuity. [23]

Increasing Unaffordability of Health Care

For most of these last 60 years, health care has been affordable for most people in this country. For those who could not pay for care, there have been safety net services available through such programs as Medicare, Medicaid, county hospitals and clinics, and providers willing to take partial payment.

The increasing escalation of prices and costs of health services, however, especially in the last 15 to 20 years, is a new phenomenon the likes of which we are yet to understand and deal with. Health care spending across the economy now exceeds 18 percent of GDP, and middle-class families' spending on health care has increased by 25 percent since 2007. [24] We have markets run amok profiteering on the backs of sick people without any effective regulation or oversight by government. Long-term care has priced itself beyond the means of most American families. Private nursing home rooms now have an annual price tag of more than $92,000. Medicare doesn't cover long-term stays, and many people have to spend down to Medicaid levels to cover needed care. [25]

Even with health insurance, many people find necessary care unaffordable. According to the 2015 Milliman Medical Index

(MMI), the cost of health insurance and care for a typical family of four with an average employer-sponsored PPO plan exceeded $25,000 in 2016, having doubled over the last ten years. [26] When you factor in forgone wage increases because of increasing costs of employer-sponsored insurance and the post-2008 recession, the affordability issue becomes desperate for so many families. Figure 6.4 shows how the essential costs of living split out for a family of four, with health care accounting for 20 percent of household income.

FIGURE 6.4

MAJOR COSTS OF LIVING FOR A FAMILY OF FOUR*

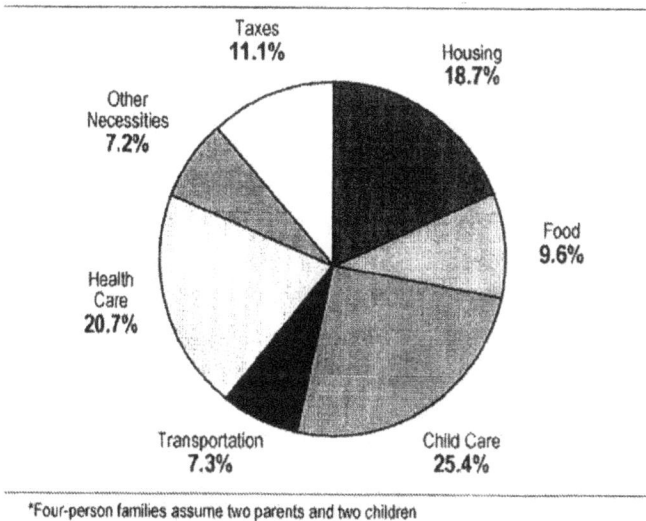

Taxes
11.1%

Housing
18.7%

Other
Necessities
7.2%

Food
9.6%

Health
Care
20.7%

Transportation
7.3%

Child Care
25.4%

*Four-person families assume two parents and two children

Source: Gould, E, Wething, H Sabadish, N et al. What Families Need to Get By: the 2013 update of EPI's Family Budget Calculator, Economics Policy Institute, Washington, D.C.

Since the median annual income for American households in 2015 was $56,500, 1.6 percent below the 2007 level, how is it possible for families to afford these high health care costs? Many can't, and this is why 1.7 million people go through bankruptcy every year because of medical bills and illness, despite most of them being middle class, owning their own homes, having attended college, and having held responsible jobs; three in four had health insurance, mostly private coverage, when they got sick. [27] Another contributing factor to medical bankruptcy is loss of income due to job loss, often because of illness. Figure 6.5 catches the irony of this critical problem.

FIGURE 6.5

POST-OP COMPLICATIONS

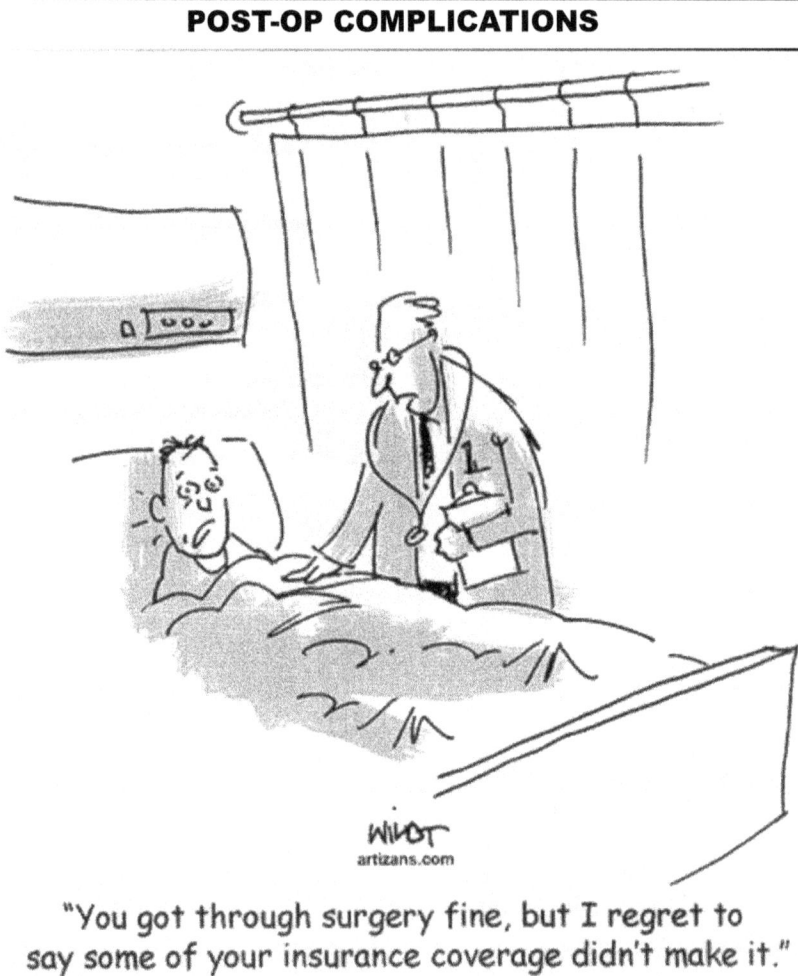

"You got through surgery fine, but I regret to say some of your insurance coverage didn't make it."

Source: Reprinted with permission of the artist, Chris Wildt

As insurers try to stay afloat, despite subsidies through the ACA, deductibles are rising rapidly. They rose by 42 percent in 2013 to an average of $5,081 a year in 2014. [28] Here is one typical patient's story that illustrates the difficult trade-off between premium affordability and exposure to out-of-pocket costs through high deductibles:

> *Edward Frank, in his 50s and looking for a job in Reynoldsville, Pennsylvania, bought a plan in late 2013 with a $6,000 deductible through the federal exchange [of the ACA]. He could not afford a plan with a lower deductible at the time. He had to pay $4,000 out of his own pocket when he needed treatment for shoulder pain. As he said, 'Unless you get desperately ill and in the hospital for weeks, it's going to cost you more to have this plan and pay the premiums than to pay the bill just outright . . . The deductibles are so high, you don't get much of anything out of it.'* [29]

Here is another common patient story that shows how unfair and morally unjust our profit-driven system has become:

> *Rosa Ines Rivera has worked as a cook in the dining halls of Harvard University's T. H. Chan School of Public Health for the last 17 years. Harvard is the country's richest university, with an endowment of some $35 billion. On the way to work every day, she sees an inscription on one of the walls that 'The highest attainable standard of health is one of the fundamental rights of every human being.' She takes home between $430 and $480 each week (approximately $24,000 a year). The administration is asking dining hall workers to pay even more for their health care*

even though some pay as much as $4,000 a year in premiums. Her premiums alone take up almost 10 percent of her income. Any actual health care costs would be financial hardship. She can no longer afford an apartment and lives with her mother and two children in public housing, with all four sharing a single bedroom. Together with 750 co-workers, she has been on strike for more affordable health care for two weeks, joined on the picket line by Harvard medical students. [30]

Drug prices for many specialty drugs are now out of sight, to the point that many patients forgo treatment. Typical yearly out-of-pocket (OOP) expenses for cancer treatment often amount to one-half of the average annual household income [31], and many cancer patients are forced to reduce the frequency of their prescribed medications and cut their spending on food and clothing in order to get by. [32] Even patients on Medicare can be hit hard by medical bills, especially for specialty drugs. Patients with cancer on Revlimid face annual payments of more than $11,000, while those with multiple sclerosis face drug bills of about $6,000 a year. [33]

According to the Commonwealth Fund Health Care Affordability Tracking Survey in late 2015, health care costs are unaffordable for 25 percent of privately insured working-age people and more than one-half of those with incomes below 200 percent of poverty ($23,340 for individuals and $47,700 for families of four).[34] A report from the Pew Charitable Trusts tells us that 55 percent of American households are so savings-limited that they can't replace less than one month of their income through liquid savings. [35] Meanwhile, overall household indebtedness has reached astronomical levels—more than $12 trillion. [36]

Failed Attempts to Control Health Care Costs

The concept that "competition" can keep prices and costs down, as it may in other industries, has long been shown by experience to not work in health care, as previously demonstrated. The health care industry is largely for-profit, minimally regulated, and is filled with perverse incentives among its stakeholders to maximize revenue. The idea that more cost-sharing with patients having more "skin in the game" has been shown to lead many patients to forgo care rather than contain costs. The non-profit Center for Studying Health System Change has studied this problem, and concluded that providers have enough market power to dictate the terms of their arrangements with insurers, and that there is insufficient competition among local health care systems. [37]

The unsuccessful results of cost containment over the last decades speak for themselves—they have not worked, as was documented in Figure 6.2. Despite its intent, this has not changed under the ACA, whether through the strategies of bundled payments, pay-for-performance (P4P), or accountable care organizations (ACOs). Quality of care measures are still too rudimentary to be useful in P4P, which are further flawed by not accounting for socio-economic determinants of patient populations, leading to inappropriate penalties of safety net hospitals and physicians practicing in poorer and disadvantaged communities. [38] ACOs, as a high-profile Medicare experiment, lack enough leverage to keep costs down, and have yet to save the government money. [39] Architects of this experimental program at Dartmouth College have recently dropped out of the program amidst increasing financial losses. [40] Wider adoption of electronic medical records, another effort by the ACA intended to improve efficiency and reduce costs, has also backfired. Instead, they have made it easier for hospitals and physicians to bill more for their services, whether appropriate or not. [41]

Trudy Lieberman, experienced journalist in health care, sums up the impact of the ACA in these words:

> *It's bad enough that the ACA is fattening up the health care industry and hollowing out coverage for the middle class. Even worse, the law is accelerating what I call the Great Cost Shift, which transfers the growing price of medical care to patients themselves through high-deductibles, coinsurance (the patient's share of the cost for a specific service, calculated as a percentage), copayments (a set fee for a specific service), and limited provider networks (which sometimes offer so little choice that patients end up seeking out-of-network care and paying on their own). What was once good, comprehensive insurance for a sizable number of Americans is being reduced to coverage for only the most serious, and most expensive of illnesses.* [42]

Concluding Comment

There are many entrenched contributors to continuing inflation of our health care costs. These include lack of any significant price controls, incentives to provide more services than we need, a prevailing business "ethic" to make as much money as possible for corporate stakeholders and their shareholders, excess capacity, and enormous levels of administrative waste. That leaves us with the highest levels of private and public spending for health care in the world. Compared to the median in other OECD countries, we even have fewer physicians, fewer nurses, fewer doctor visits, fewer hospital beds, and fewer hospital days per capita. [43] The most important reason for these differences is the lack of accountability in our free-wheeling profit-driven system.

In the next chapter, we will look at another way that patients lose out in our present system by not being able to afford and get essential health care.

Endnotes:

1. Berwick, D. A transatlantic review of the NHS at 60. *British Medical Journal* 337 (7663): 212-214, 2008.

2. Geyman, JP. *Health Care in America: Can Our Ailing System Be Healed?* Woburn, MA. *Butterworth-Heinemann*, 2002, p. 94.

3. Keehan, SP, Cuckler, GA, Sisko, AM et al. National health expenditure projections, 2014-2024: Spending growth faster than recent trends. *Health Affairs on line*, July 28, 2015.

4. Johnson, C. By 2024, health spending will be nearly a fifth of the economy. *The Washington Post*, July 28, 2015.

5. Calculation using Dr. Petrosino's Education Project. February 17, 2016.

6. Alonso-Zaldivar, R. Health. $10,345 per person: U.S. health care spending reaches new peak. *Associated Press*, July 16, 2016.

7. Radnofsky, L. Insurers seek big premium boosts. *Wall Street Journal*, May 26, 2016: B1.

8. Neprash, HT, Chernew, ME, Hicks, AL et al. Association of financial integration with commercial health care prices. *JAMA Internal Medicine*, October 19, 2015.

9. Dickson, V. Blog: Doctors say Medicare pays three times more for care in hospital outpatient departments. *Modern Health Care*, February 18, 2016.

10. Rabin, RC. How much to deliver a baby? Charges vary widely by hospital. *KHN Blog*, January 16, 2014.

11. Jaffe, S. FAQ: Hospital observation care can be poorly understood and costly for Medicare beneficiaries. *Kaiser Health News*, September 4, 2013.

12. Mathews, AW, Weaver, C. Study: Patient discharges tied to payments. *Wall Street Journal*, June 9, 2015.

13. Himmelstein, DU, Jun, M, Busse, R et al. A comparison of hospital administrative costs in eight nations: U.S. costs exceed all others by far. *Health Affairs*, September 2014.

14. Loftus, P. Ads for costly drugs get airtime. *Wall Street Journal*, February 17, 2016: B1.

15. Johnson, LA. Teva offers to buy Mylan in $40.1 billion cash-and-stock deal. *ABC News*, April 15, 2015.

16. Rosenthal, E. Officials question the rising costs of generic drugs. *New York Times*, October 7, 2014.

17. Berkrot, B. Number of Americans using $100,000 in medicines triples – Express Scripts. *Reuters*, May 13, 2015.

18. Whalen, J. U.S. drug prices dwarf other nations. *Wall Street Journal*, December 1, 2015.

19. Blackwell, R. Drug prices expected to rise as result of TPP deal. *The Globe and Mail*, December 6, 2015.

20. Bulik, BS. Pharmacists join physicians' rallying cry for a ban on pharma's DTC advertising. *Fierce Pharma,* June 20, 2016.

21. Austin, DR, Baker, LC. Less physician practice competition is associated with higher prices paid for common procedures. *Health Affairs* 34 (10): 1753-1760, 2015.

22. Rosenthal, E. Patients' costs skyrocket; specialists' incomes soar. *New York Times*, January 18, 2014.

23. Rosenthal, E. As insurers try to limit costs, providers hit patients with more separate fees. *New York Times*, October 25, 2014.

24. Sussman, AL. Health burden moves to the middle. *Wall Street Journal,* August 26, 2016: A2.

25. Associated Press. Study: Costs for most long-term care keep climbing. *New York Times,* May 10, 2016.

26. Milliman. 2015 Milliman Medical Index. May 2015.

27. Himmelstein, DU, Thorne, D, Warren, E. et al. Medical bankruptcy in the United States, 2007: results of a national study. *Amer J Med* 122 (8): 741-746, 2009.

28. Scism, L, Martin, TW. Deductibles fuel new worries of health-law sticker shock. *Wall Street Journal*, December 9, 2013.

29. *Associated Press*. Health care insecurity. Poll: many insured struggle with medical bills. October 13, 2014.

30. Rivera, RI. Struggling to serve at the nation's richest university. *New York Times*, October 24, 2016.

31. Kantarjian, J, Steensma, D, San Juan, JR et al. High cancer drug prices in the United States: Reasons and proposed solutions. *J Oncology Practice*, May 6, 2014.

32. Zafarm, SY, Peppercorn, JM, Schrag, D et al. The financial toxicity of cancer treatment: a pilot study assessing out-of-pocket expenses and the insured cancer patient's experience. *Oncologist* 18: 381-390, 2013.

33. Walker, J. Drug prices jolt middle class. *Wall Street Journal*, January 23, 2016: A 1.

34. How high is America's health care cost burden? Findings from the Commonwealth Fund Health Care Affordability Tracking Survey, July-August 2015. Issue Brief. *The Commonwealth Fund.* November 20, 2015.

35. The precarious state of family balance sheets. *Pew Charitable Trusts*, January 29, 2015.

36. Zumbrun, J. Baby boomers pile on the debt. *Wall Street Journal*, February 13-14, 2016.

37. Nichols, LM et al. Are market forces strong enough to deliver efficient health care systems? Confidence is waning. *Health Affairs* 23 (2): 8-21, 2004.

38. Ryan, J, Doty, MM, Hamel, L et al. Primary care providers' views of trends in health care delivery and payment. *The Commonwealth Fund and the Kaiser Family Foundation*, August 5, 2015.

39. Rau, J, Gold, J. Medicare yet to save money through heralded medical payment model. *Kaiser Health News*, September 14, 2015.

40. Pear, R. Dropout by Dartmouth raises questions on health law cost-savings effort. *New York Times*, September 10, 2016.

41. Abelson, R, Creswell, J, Palmer, G. Medicare bills rise as records turn electronic. *New York Times,* September 22, 2012.

42. Lieberman, T. Wrong prescription? The failed promise of the Affordable Care Act. *Harper's Magazine*, July 2015.

43. Squires, D, Anderson, C. U.S. health care from a global perspective: Spending, use of services, prices, and health in 13 countries. *The Commonwealth Fund*, October 8, 2015.

CHAPTER 7

DECREASED ACCESS
AND QUALITY OF CARE

All of the trends in the last six chapters—increasing specialization, decline of primary care, increasing technology, corporatization, increasing privatization, soaring costs and unaffordability of
care—are intertwined in reducing both access and quality of care.
When people can't gain access to care for financial or other reasons,
they tend to forgo necessary care and have worse outcomes if and
when they finally get care. In essence, there can't be good quality of
care without ready access to care

This chapter has three goals: (1) to look at what has happened
to access to health care before and over the last 60 years; (2) to discuss more recent factors that have reduced the quality of care; and
(3) to compare quality of care by state and internationally.

Access to Care: Historical Perspective

The Great Depression, starting in 1929 but extending through the
1930s, had a severe impact on medical care throughout the country. In response, a not-for-profit health insurance industry began to
emerge and the federal government became involved in health care
for the first time. The Committee on the Costs of Medical Care
(CCMC) made these important recommendations in 1932, all still
relevant today:

1. Medical service should be furnished largely by organized groups.

2. Basic public health services should be extended so they will be available to the entire population according to its needs.

3. The costs of medical care should be placed on a group payment basis through the use of insurance or taxation or both. [1]

In 1935, as part of President Franklin D. Roosevelt's New Deal, the Social Security Act was passed, together with federal funds to local health departments for maternal and child health services. [2]

Blue Cross and Blue Shield established the first private health insurance plans in the 1930s, which provided discounted rates for hospitals and physicians whereby more people could afford care with minimal out-of-pocket payments and hospital beds were kept open. [3]

Voluntary health insurance grew rapidly after World War II, especially for the employed and their dependents, facilitated by its tax-exempt status to employers. [4] By the 1960s there were widespread concerns about access to care, especially among the elderly and poor. In response, Medicare and Medicaid were enacted in 1965, which led to growth in the number of physicians and hospital beds as well as the start of health care inflation. Federal projections at the time estimated a $10 billion outlay for Medicare in 1990, just 10 percent of what it turned out to be. [5]

During my practice years in the 1960s, patients had good access to care, especially after the passage of Medicare and Medicaid, with full choice of physician and hospital. Affordability was a problem for many patients, but physicians and hospitals would generally accept the care of everyone who was sick, with arrangements for dealing with payment on a sliding scale or charity basis.

The major concern in the 1960s was access to care, which shifted to costs by the 1990s, when managed care came along as a supposed solution, as we will discuss in Chapter 13. The insurance industry rolled out their low-premium, high-deductible "consumer directed health plans," a strategy giving insurers a stable revenue source while forcing many enrollees to forgo care because of uncovered costs. [6] That trend has persisted over the last 20 years, though the details have changed.

Decreasing Access to Care since 2010

In response to 50 million Americans being uninsured and many more underinsured, the 2010 Affordable Care Act (ACA) attempted to address these problems, but its results after six years has been a mixed report. On the one hand, at least 16 million people have gained insurance either through state or federal exchanges or through expansion of Medicaid. The ACA enacted some restraints on insurers, such as not being able to exclude enrollees based on pre-existing conditions and allowing parents to keep their children on their policies until age 26. But, despite these gains, these are some of the ongoing problems still unresolved in 2017:

- There are still 28 million Americans uninsured [7] and more than 30 million underinsured.
- 19 states refused to expand Medicaid, and there is a "Medicaid coverage gap" affecting 4.8 million people who earn too much to qualify for insurance through the exchanges and too little to qualify for existing Medicaid. Dr. Jack Geiger, a founder of the community health center model, had this to say about this predicament:

> *The irony is that these states that are rejecting Medicaid expansion—many of them Southern—are the very places where the concentration of poverty and lack of health insurance are the most acute. It is their populations that have the highest burden of illness and costs to the entire health care system.* [8]

- Because of poor reimbursement to physicians (about 61 percent of what insurers pay for private coverage), only two-thirds of primary care physicians nationally will see new patients on Medicaid. [9]. Restricted access to non-primary care specialists is a more serious barrier for Medicaid patients with long waiting times if they ever can find a specialist to see them. A 2014 study found that most patients newly covered by Medicaid expansion under the ACA are in private managed care plans in which one-half of physicians do not accept new Medicaid patients or are unavailable at their last known address. [10] Figure 7.1 shows how difficult it is for Medicaid patients to see primary care physicians for after-hours care.

FIGURE 7.1

ACCESS TO AFTER-HOURS PRIMARY CARE

Primary care physicians, 2012
Practice has arrangement for patients'
after-hours care to see doctor or nurse

Percent

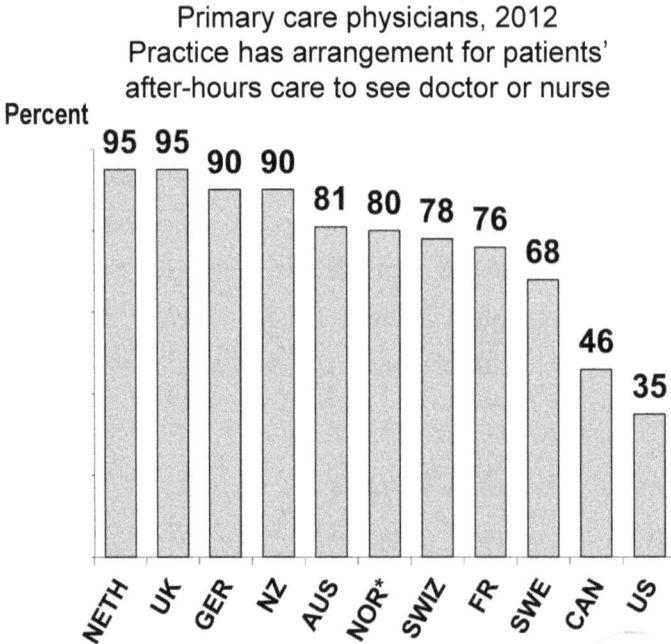

Source: Osborn, R, Schoen, C. 2013 International Health Policy Survey in Eleven Countries. *The Commonwealth Fund*, November 2013. Reprinted with permission.

- California, with more than 13 million enrollees on Medi-Cal, its Medicaid program, and some of the lowest Medicaid provider payment rates in the country, has great difficulty gaining access to care for these patients in public safety net facilities, even including San Francisco General Hospital and Harbor-UCLA Medical Center. [11]

- Some states, such as Texas, Ohio, and Colorado, have opened for-profit, freestanding emergency departments in more affluent zip code areas, which are exempt from federal requirements that protect patients in hospital ERs from being denied care if they can't afford it. [12].

- Insurer networks are constantly changing, based on negotiated costs and not quality, disrupting continuity of care and often forcing patients to change networks.

- Waiting times vary widely by specialty and from one part of the country to another; as examples, wait times to see a dermatologist in 2014 averaged 29 days, 66 days to get a physical examination in Boston, and 32 days for a heart evaluation by a cardiologist in Washington, D.C. [13]

- The ACA's accountable care organizations are another way of limiting patients' access and continuity of care, even when insured; here is one example—UnitedHealth Group, the biggest player in the Medicare Advantage market with almost 3 million enrollees and 350,000 physicians in its networks, dropped thousands of physicians from its networks in at least ten states in the last months of 2013, forcing about 2,500 cancer patients at Moffitt Cancer Center in Tampa, Florida, to switch plans or find other physicians. [14]

- A recent study by the Inspector General of the Department of Health and Human Services found that one-half of physicians listed as serving Medicaid patients are unavailable or unable to make appointments. [15]

Decreasing Quality of Care

Let's look at four factors that reduce the quality of care that Americans receive.

1. Insurance coverage matters.

It is logical and has been documented many times that the insured receive better quality of care than the uninsured, but there are differences in the value of insurance. We also know that people on Medicaid do better than those without Medicaid, but here again there are big differences in the value of coverage from state to state. Then there are differences in the quality of coverage when public Medicare and Medicaid programs are compared with their privatized counterparts. Here are examples that show some of these differences:

- According to 2012 estimates by Harvard researchers and the U.S. Census Bureau, 50,000 Americans were dying each year for lack of health insurance—136 per day—when there were 50 million uninsured; that estimate today under the ACA is about 28,000 annual deaths.[16]

- Among the "insured", there are many policies marketed, even meeting ACA requirements, that give poor coverage, such as policies that last less than one year or minimal coverage of specialty drugs that might force some cancer patients to forgo recommended treatment.

- The quality of care received by insured patients *within the same hospital* can vary, with Medicare patients getting worse care than those with private coverage. [17]

- Privatized Medicare plans tend to have worse outcomes than traditional public Medicare, especially for sick patients [18], and the same difference also applies to privatized Medicaid. [19]

- Medicaid generally gives better coverage and outcomes than being uninsured, as was shown in Oregon [20], but eligibility and coverage of Medicaid varies widely from one state to another.

- It is estimated that 7,115 to 17,104 unnecessary deaths will be attributable to the refusal of 20 states to expand Medicaid under the ACA. [21]

2. Overutilization

- Up to one-third of all health care services provided in the U.S. are unnecessary or inappropriate, and some are actually harmful [22]; one example is the overuse of elective cardiac catheterization, which carries significant risk. [23]
- The American Board of Internal Medicine has recently found that three of four physicians surveyed believe that unnecessary tests and procedures are a serious problem. [24]
- Polypharmacy is a common problem among older adults who see multiple physicians, who do not talk to each other, for chronic problems; 40 percent take five or more prescription drugs while 18 percent take ten or more. [25]

3. Lack of coordination.

- Lack of communication within our fragmented, over-specialized system leads to worse quality of care, as this 2010 Report from the Josiah Macy, Jr. Foundation made clear:

> *Too often, patients with acute or chronic health conditions receive services from multiple health providers in multiple care settings that do not coordinate and communicate with each other. This is especially true for the vulnerable elderly and disabled populations. This lack of coordination and integration leads to a fragmented healthcare system in which patients experience questionable care with more errors, more waste and duplication, and little accountability for quality and cost efficiency.* [26]

- Excessive prescribing by multiple physicians not communicating with each other—polypharmacy—is a common problem caused by fragmentation of care among specialists; it accounts for drug-related complications among more than one-half hospitalized elderly patients.[27]

4. For profit facilities, especially when investor-owned, have lower quality of care compared to their not-for-profit counterparts.

- Hospitals: Costs higher, fewer nurses, and higher death rates[28]
- Rehabilitation hospitals: Almost one-third of patients in these facilities suffer preventable medication errors, bedsores, infection, or other harms as a result of their care. [29]
- Nursing homes: Lower staffing levels and worse quality of care[30]
- Mental health centers: Restrictive barriers and limits to care [31]
- Dialysis centers: higher hospitalization rates [32]
- Home health agencies: Higher costs, lower quality of care [33]

In response to these major problems in quality of care in this country, have any of our system responses worked to improve quality, whether accountable care organizations, pay-for-performance (P4P), or the National Committee for Quality Assurance (NCQA)? These observations by two leaders in this field give us no such assurance:

> *An exhaustive study by the Cochrane collaborative, an international group that reviews medical evidence, unearthed 'no evidence that financial incentives can improve patient outcomes' . . . One Boston area hospital we ob-*

served improved its quality score 40 percent just by getting doctors to change the words they wrote in patients' charts.

Medicare gives hospitals more credit for saving patients with "acute respiratory decompensation" than those with "COPD exacerbations," although these terms are synonymous. That kind of practice is neither illegal nor unusual. [34]

—Dr. Steffie Woolhandler, internist
and health policy expert

My main gripe now is what I see as contradictory strategies of high deductibles versus a delivery system reform promoting primary care. If you spend out of your own pocket $2,000 or $5,000 before you get to see your primary care physician (for free), many Americans don't have that money. We are reforming the delivery system and then people can't afford to see their primary care doctor. That makes no sense. [35]

—Margaret "Peggy" O'Kane, founding and current president of
the National Committee for Quality Assurance (NCQA)

Medicare's new five-star rating system has already proven itself of little value as it over-values relatively obscure hospitals that specialize in a few surgical procedures for more affluent patients while down-grading many highly acclaimed hospitals, typically teaching hospitals, and ignoring socio-economic factors that adversely affect their lower-income patient populations. [36]

State and International Comparisons of Quality of Care

We all know that quality of care can be elusive, and that no health care system is perfect, but how do we compare across the country by state and with other advanced countries? Fortunately, this has been well studied, but the results are not encouraging.

The Commonwealth Fund has conducted studies of all 50 states and the District of Columbia for the last four years, measuring and ranking states in five domains—access and affordability, prevention and treatment, avoidable hospital use and costs, healthy lives, and equity. Wide variations have been found, with up to an eight-fold difference between top- and bottom-ranked states on some measures. There are big regional differences in overall performance of states' health care systems, with the best-performing states clustered in the Northeast and Upper Midwest, as shown in Figure 7.2. Overall, more states improved than worsened in the 2015 report. [37]

Cross-national comparisons also leave much to be desired. Here again, the Commonwealth Fund has provided us with the best available information. The U.S. is again an outlier among 11 advanced countries by quality of care as measured by mortality amenable to health care. While some improvement occurred between 1997-1998 and 2006-2007, the U.S. still had the highest number of deaths per 100,000 population, nearly double that of France. (Figure 7.3) [38]

Concluding Comment

As the above makes clear, we are far from having the best health care system in the world. We have to overcome this myth and look hard at the evidence that shows us how far we need to go before we can say that we are meeting the needs of our population for affordable, quality health care. We need to take a broader view of the challenge, realizing that health care reform to date has failed and that access, cost, and quality of health care are intertwined and interdependent. This insight from Dr. Aaron Carroll, professor of pediatrics and director of the Center for Health Policy and Professionalism at Indiana University School of Medicine, is right on target:

One of the most important facts about health care overhaul, and one that is often overlooked, is that all changes to the health system involve trade-offs among access, quality and cost. You can improve one of these— maybe two—but it will always result in some other aspect getting worse. [As examples] you can make the health care system achieve better outcomes. But that will usually cost more or require some change in access. You can make it cheaper, but access or quality may take a hit. [39]

Decreased Access and Quality of Care

FIGURE 7.2

HIGHLIGHTS FROM THE STATES' SCORECARD

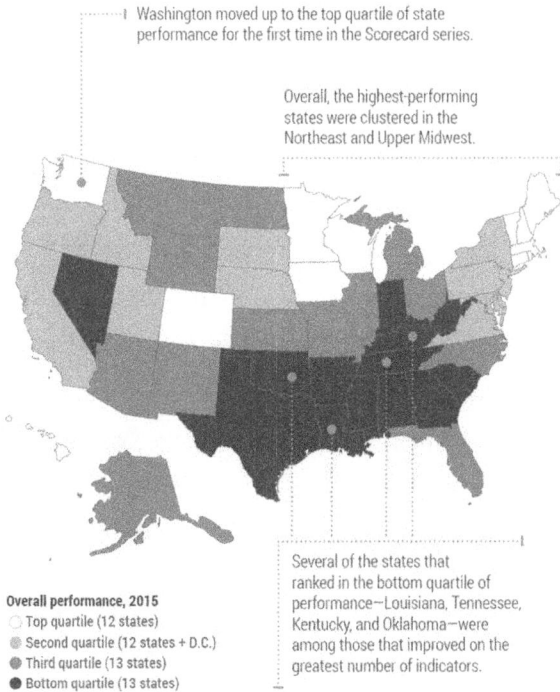

Washington moved up to the top quartile of state performance for the first time in the Scorecard series.

Overall, the highest-performing states were clustered in the Northeast and Upper Midwest.

Several of the states that ranked in the bottom quartile of performance—Louisiana, Tennessee, Kentucky, and Oklahoma—were among those that improved on the greatest number of indicators.

Overall performance, 2015
- Top quartile (12 states)
- Second quartile (12 states + D.C.)
- Third quartile (13 states)
- Bottom quartile (13 states)

Source: McCarthy, D, Radley, DC, Hayes, SL. Results from scorecard on state health system performance, December, 2015 *The Commonwealth Fund.* Reprinted with permission.

FIGURE 7.3

CROSS NATIONAL COMPARISON OF MORTALITY AMENABLE TO HEALTH CARE

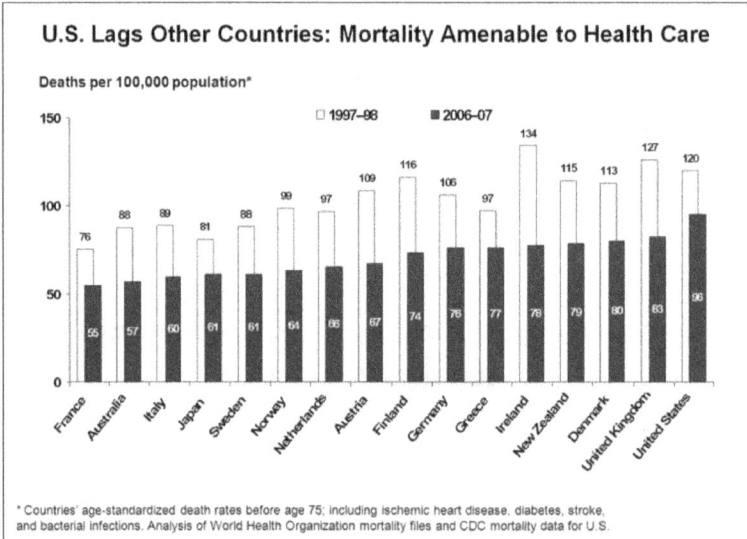

U.S. Lags Other Countries: Mortality Amenable to Health Care

Deaths per 100,000 population*

□ 1997–98   ■ 2006–07

Country	1997–98	2006–07
France	76	55
Australia	88	57
Italy	89	60
Japan	81	61
Sweden	88	61
Norway	99	64
Netherlands	97	66
Austria	109	67
Finland	116	74
Germany	106	76
Greece	97	77
Ireland	134	78
New Zealand	115	79
Denmark	113	80
United Kingdom	127	83
United States	120	96

* Countries' age-standardized death rates before age 75; including ischemic heart disease, diabetes, stroke, and bacterial infections. Analysis of World Health Organization mortality files and CDC mortality data for U.S.

Source: The Commonwealth Fund. Reprinted with permission.

We need to recognize and deal with these trade-offs and be willing to address them politically in the public interest. In the meantime, until we get more proactive about fundamental health care reform, individuals, their families, and the nation suffers from less access to quality health care and a worse system than we pay for or deserve.

Endnotes:

1. Falk, IS. Some lessons from the fifty years since the COMC Final Report, 1932. *J Public Health Policy* 4 (2): 139, 1983.

2. Rosenblatt, RA, Moscovice, IS. *Rural Health Care.* New York. *John Wiley*, 1982, p. 33.

3. McNerney, W. C. Rufus Rorem award lecture. Big question for the Blues: Where to go from here? *Inquiry* (Summer) 33: 110-117, 1983.

4. Somers, AR, Somers, HM. *Health and Health Care: Policies in Perspective.* Germantown, MD. *Aspen Systems Corp.*, 1977.

5. Ginsburg, E. Ten encounters with the U.S. health sector: 1930-1999. *JAMA* 282: 1665-1668. 1999.

6. Altman, D. Covering the uninsured: Not just a red state issue. *Wall Street Journal*, October 14, 2015.

7. Potter, W. Insurers' high-deductible plans leave Americans without needed care. *The Progressive Populist*, June 15, 2015, p. 15.

8. Geiger, J. As cited by Tavernise, S, Gebeloff, R. Millions of poor are left uncovered by health law. *New York Times*, October 2, 2013.

9. Decker, SL. Two-thirds of primary care physicians accepted new Medicaid patients in 2011-2012: A baseline to measure future acceptance rates. *Health Affairs* 32 (7): 1183-1187, 2013.

10. Pear, R Half of doctors listed as serving Medicaid patients are unavailable, investigation finds. *New York Times*, December 8, 2014.

11. Bartolone, P. California's public hospitals face new Medi-Cal mandate. *California Healthline*, August 4, 2016.

12. Schuur, JD, Baker, O, Freshman, J et al. Where do freestanding emergency departments choose to locate? A national inventory and geographic analysis in three states. *Annals of Emergency Medicine*, July 12, 2016 (online).

13. Rosenthal, E. The health care waiting game: Long waits for doctors' appointments have become the norm. *New York Times*, July 5, 2014.

14. Beck, M. United Health culls doctors from plan. *Wall Street Journal*, November 16, 2013: B1.

15. Pear, R. Half of doctors listed as serving Medicaid patients are unavailable, investigation finds. *New York Times*, December 8, 2014.

16. Wolfe, S. Outrage of the Month! 50 million uninsured in the U.S. equals 50,000+ avoidable deaths each year. *Health Letter* 28 (1): 11, January 2012.

17. Spencer, CS, Gaskin, DJ, Roberts, ET. The quality of care delivered to patients within the same hospital varies by insurance type. *Health Affairs* 32 (10): 1731-1739, 2013.

18. Gold, M, Casillas, G. What do we know about health care access and quality in Medicare Advantage versus the traditional Medicare program? *Kaiser Family Foundation*, November 6, 2014.

19. McCue, MJ, Bailit, MH. Assessing the financial health of Medicaid managed care plans and the quality of care they provide. New York. *The Commonwealth Fund*, June 15, 2011.

20. Baicker, K, Taubman, SL, Allen, HL et al. The Oregon experiment—effects of Medicaid on clinical outcomes. *N Engl J Med* 368 (18): 1713-1722, May 2, 2013.

21. Dickman, S et al. Opting out of Medicaid expansion: The health and financial impacts. *Health Affairs Blog*, January 30, 2014.

22. Wenner, JB, Fisher, ES, Skinner, JS. Geography and the debate over Medicare reform. *Health Affairs Web Exclusive* W-103, February 13, 2002.

23. Patel, MR, Peterson, ED, Dai, MS et al. Low diagnostic yield of elective coronary angiography. *N Engl J Med* 362: 862-895, 2010.

24. Hancock, J. How tiny are benefits from many tests and pills? Researchers paint a picture. *Kaiser Health News*, October 12, 2016.

25. Landro, L. Medication overload. *Wall Street Journal*, October 1, 2016: D1.

26. Mitchener, JL, Berkowitz, B, Aguilar-Gaaxiola, S et al. Designing new models of care for diverse communities: Why new modes of care delivery are needed. In Cronenwett, L, Dzau, V, Culliton, B, Russell, S (eds) *Who Will Provide Primary Care and How Will They Be Trained?* Proceedings of a conference sponsored by the Josiah Macy, Jr., Foundation, Durham, NC 2010, pp. 84-85.

27. Gorman, A. 'America's other drug problem': Copious prescriptions for hospitalized elderly. *Kaiser Health News*, August 30, 2016.

28. Yuan, Z, Cooper, GS, Einstadter, D et al. The association between hospital type and mortality and length of stay: A study of 16.9 million hospitalized Medicare beneficiaries. *Medical Care* 38: 231, 2000.

29. Allen, M. New report: Problem care harms almost one-third of rehab hospital patients. *ProPublica*, July 21, 2016.

30. Harrington, C, Woolhandler, S, Mullen, J et al. Does investor-ownership of nursing homes compromise the quality of care? *Amer J Public Health* 91 (9): 1, 2001.

31. Munoz, R. How health care insurers avoid treating mental illness. *San Diego Union Tribune*, May 22, 2002.

32. Dalrymple, LS, Johansen, KL, Romano, PS et al. Comparison of hospitalization rates among for-profit and non-profit dialysis facilities. *Clinical Journal of the American Society of Nephrology.* 9 (1): 73-81, 2014.

33. Cabin, W, Himmelstein, DU, Siman, ML et al. For-profit Medicare home health agencies' costs appear higher and quality appears lower compared to non-profit agencies. *Health Affairs* 33 (8):1460-1465, 2014.

34. Woolhandler, S. Should physician pay be tied to performance? No, the system is too easy to game—and too hard to set up. *Wall Street Journal*, June 16, 2013.

35. O'Kane, M. As quoted by Galewitz, P. Health plan watchdog still seeks progress after 25 years. *Kaiser Health News*, January 8, 2016.

36. Rau, J. Many well-known hospitals fail to score 5 stars in Medicare's new ratings. *Kaiser Health News*, July 27, 2016.

37. McCarthy, D, Radley, DC, Hayes, SL. *Aiming Higher: Results from a Scorecard on State Health System Performance*, 2015 edition, December 9, 2015.

38. Osborn, R, Moulds, D. *The Commonwealth Fund 2014 International Health Policy Survey of Older Adults in Eleven Countries*, November 2014, p. 20.

39. Carroll, AE. Why improving access to health care does not save money. *New York Times*, July 14, 2014.

CHAPTER 8

DEPERSONALIZATION OF HEALTH CARE

It has been sad to see how health care has become so depersonalized. Sixty years ago, the first question a physician or receptionist would ask of the patient was: "What can I (or we) do for you today?" (I learned early on not to ask "What brought you here today?" after getting the response "My 51 Chevy, of course!") Today, the first questions asked in any medical office are "What is your insurance?" and "Your birth date, please?"

We learned throughout medical school in the 1950s that the patient's story—the history—will usually give you the diagnosis if you listen well enough. Today, there is little time for history as so many physicians jump to laboratory tests and imaging procedures, typically while looking at a computer screen instead of the patient's face.

This chapter has two goals: (1) to discuss ten inter-related trends that have depersonalized health care, altered the doctor-patient relationship, and diminished the personhood of the patient; and (2) to briefly consider the impacts of these changes on the healing process.

Ten Trends toward Depersonalization of Health Care
1. Increasing specialization and changing doctor-patient relationship

As we saw in Chapters 4 and 5, the proportion of generalist physicians more than reversed between 1930, when 80 percent were generalists, to less than 20 percent in 2016. Medicine has broken into some 150 specialties and sub-specialties, each concerned with a smaller part of the whole patient, and often not communicating among themselves. House calls, which I always found so rewarding during my Mount Shasta years in learning more about the patient, his or her family, their circumstances and values, are virtually a relic of the past. That knowledge of the patient is not gained in short office visits, and is so necessary to understanding how to deal with challenging medical decisions, such as in serious illness and end-of-life care.

At the opposite extreme today, and hopefully not an increasing trend, is a recent report that WellPoint and Aetna, two insurance giants, are allowing millions of patients to have first visits by e-mail with their physicians "in order to cut costs and diagnose minor ailments." Such visits decrease what often needs to be learned by careful history combined with physical examination. These insurers are joining with other companies, such as Teladoc, MDLive, and American Well that offer virtual visits with physicians who, in some states, can prescribe drugs for conditions ranging from back pain to sinus infections. This trend, pushed by insurers and the companies so involved, remains controversial within the profession, and is an active issue for state licensing policies and state medical boards. [1]

To be fair, there is another side to the use of e-mail between patients and physicians. We have seen a trend for some time toward concierge medicine, whereby patients have an established relationship over time with a primary care physician, which includes the appropriate use of e-mail. But national companies with physicians who never see the patient, except online, are another matter, with risk to the patient of misdiagnosis and inappropriate treatment without understanding the patient's story. [2]

2. *Reimbursement favoring procedures and lab/imaging tests, less talk and listening*

The long-standing Resource Based Relative Value Scale (RBRVS) system for reimbursement of physicians' services has from the beginning favored the value of surgical and diagnostic procedures over more time-intensive services, such as the talking and listening so important in the primary care specialties, geriatrics, and psychiatry. The main mechanism of setting these values under the fee-for-service system—the AMA's Relative Value Scale Update Committee (RUC)—is full of conflicts of interest. Its 29 representatives are mostly selected by medical specialty societies, with little representation of the primary care specialties. Predictably, each specialty society has a vested interest in gaining maximal reimbursement for its services. RUC's recommendations are generally followed by CMS, which has no authority to re-adjust overvalued billing codes, which are pervasive throughout the system. One example is a billing code that pays podiatrists more than $3,100 for treating a foot ulcer with the skin substitute Dermagraft. [3]

3. *Corporatization and efficiency*

As we saw in Chapter 1, most physicians today are under pressure to be "more productive," meaning seeing more patients in a shorter amount of time, and providing more volume of billable services. Time has become money, and so often physicians' jobs depend on how they adapt to their employers' expectations for revenue. A physician or other health care professional is not "efficient" when he or she spends 45 minutes taking a more lengthy history that can help to more accurately make a diagnosis as well as better understand the patient's story, needs, and values.

4. *Narrow and changing networks*

Narrow networks have become endemic under the ACA, which permits insurers to exclude almost one-third of "essential community providers," often so narrow that such specialists as endocrinologists, rheumatologists, and psychiatrists are not included. [4] Patients end up as pawns in the ongoing negotiations between insurers, hospitals and physician groups over networks. These negotiations, of course, are about money, not about what's best for patients. Insurers want to get the lowest costs in order to offer lower premiums and attract more enrollees. Hospitals are seeking to maximize their reimbursements, as are physician groups. Patients often find that their networks of physicians and hospitals have changed, and many directories of network physicians are inaccurate when they try to change physicians. [5]

5. *Less continuity of care*

Continuity of care over years, especially with a primary care physician, has been and should be the foundation of the doctor-patient relationship, facilitating coordination of care when other physicians and providers are involved. But under the guise of "competition" and "efficiency," continuity of care has been disrupted for many patients throughout the system. The ACA has accelerated that process through mergers and consolidation among hospital systems, business decisions of insurers, and instability created by accountable care organizations. A 2013 example shows how sudden and disruptive this trend can be when several hundred patients at the University of Pittsburgh Medical Center (UPMC) received certified letters informing them that they could no longer see their physicians. Their insurer, Community Blue, sold by Highmark, had become both a rival hospital system and an insurer. Cancer patients were cut off from their UPMC physicians even in the middle of their therapy. [6]

As a result of the primary care shortage, first-visits are increasingly being made to drugstore, grocery store clinics, or other retailers such as Target Corp., especially for minor illnesses and problems not of an emergency nature. Such clinics provide convenience care without any continuity. [7] The rapid growth of virtual visits through telemedicine further disrupts continuity of care. Fifteen million Americans received some kind of care this way in 2015, according to the American Telemedicine Association, which expects this number to grow by 30 percent in 2016. [8]

6. *Split of hospital care from outpatient care*

Sixty years ago, it was a norm that the physician admitting a patient into the hospital would follow and continue the patient's care there, with or without calling in other physicians as consultants. That practice has withered over the years, partly again in the name of efficiency—allowing the physician to see more patients in the office. Today, hospitalists, typically unknown previously to patients, play a coordinative role during a patient's hospitalization, but usually without involvement with the patient's primary care physician (if he or she has one). The result is often chaotic, with frequent miscommunication among specialists, uninformed by the patient's narrative that should influence his or her treatment. As Dr. Arnold Relman observed after a terrible ordeal breaking his neck in a fall:

> *What is important is that someone who knows the patient oversees their care, ensures that the many specialized services work together in the patient's interest, and that the patient is fully involved and informed. . . . The growing national shortage of primary care physicians allows for fragmentation, duplication, and lack of coordination of medical services.* [9]

7. *Physicians as employees under "production pressures"*

Self-employed physicians in solo or small-group practice, the norm 60 years ago, are almost extinct today. Nearly two-thirds of practicing physicians are now employed by large hospital systems, some even by insurers. As employees, physicians have lost much of their past clinical autonomy, are under pressure to be "more productive," as determined by their non-physician masters. Not surprisingly, they increasingly complain of less practice satisfaction. This observation by Dr. David Eddy, well-known expert in clinical decision making and author of the landmark book, *Clinical Decision Making: From Theory to Practice*, written 20 years ago, shows how inexorable the trends since then have transformed today's medical practice:

> *Medical practice is in the middle of a profound transition. Most physicians can remember the day when, armed with a degree, a mission, and confidence, they could set forth to heal the sick. Like Solomon, physicians could receive patients, hear their complaints and determine the best course of action. While not every patient could be cured, everyone could be confident that whatever was done was the best possible. Most important, each physician was free, trusted, and left alone to determine what was in the best interest of each patient.*

> *All of that is changing. In retrospect, the first changes seem minor—some increased paperwork, "tissue" committees, a few more meetings. These activities were designed to affect the presumably small fraction of physicians who, in fact, deserved to be scrutinized, and the scrutiny was an internal process performed by physicians themselves. But today's activities are aimed at all physicians, are much more anonymous, and seem beyond physician control. Now*

physicians must deal with second opinions, precertifica-
tion, skeptical medical directors, variable coverage, out-
right denials, utilization review, threats of cookbook medi-
cine, and letters out of the blue chiding that Mrs. Smith is
on two incompatible drugs. Solomon did not have to call
anyone to get permission for his decisions. [10]

8. *Health care as a commodity*

As we have seen in earlier chapters, U.S. health care, as a medical-industrial complex, has become big business, with ever-larger corporate stakeholders vying for profits for themselves and their Wall Street shareholders. Health care has become a commodity for sale on a largely deregulated market. Dr. Edmund Pellegrino, as a leading medical ethicist at Georgetown University's Center for Clinical Bioethics, warned his fellow physicians in 1990 of what has come to pass:

> *Medicine is at heart a moral enterprise and those who*
> *practice it are de facto members of a moral community.*
> *We can accept or repudiate that fact, but we cannot ignore*
> *it or absolve ourselves of the moral consequences of our*
> *choice. We are not a guild, business, trade union, or a po-*
> *litical party. If the care of the sick is increasingly treated as*
> *a commodity, and investment opportunity, a bureaucrat's*
> *power trip, or a political trading chip, the profession bears*
> *part of the responsibility.* [11]

9. *Business "ethic" replacing service ethic*

We will discuss this in more detail in the next chapter, but for now this observation by Dr. Albert Jonsen, bioethicist and former chairman of the University of Washington's Department of Medical History and Ethics, is spot on:

The encounter between patient and physician is no longer a private place. It is a cubicle with open walls, surrounded by a crowd of managers, regulators, financiers, producers and lawyers required to manage the flow of money that makes the encounter possible. All of them can look into the encounter and see opportunities for profit or economy. All would like to have a say in how the encounter goes—from the time consumed by it, to the drugs prescribed in it, to the costing out of each of its elements. [12]

10. *Patient narratives lost in electronic medical records*

The ACA brought new emphasis and funding for wider adoption of electronic health records (EHRs) based on an assumption that they would improve communication, patient safety, efficiency, reduce diagnostic testing, and save money. The opposite has happened. Instead, EHRs have been used mainly for billing purposes (facilitating up-coding for reimbursement purposes), have raised costs, [13] and reduced efficiency. Competing systems do not talk to each other. Templates that go into the records typically have much non-relevant information and completely exclude the patient's narrative. EHRs actually intrude into the doctor-patient relationship as physicians (or increasingly, their scribes) put more attention on the record than the patient. A 2013 report from the RAND Corporation drew these conclusions, among others:

- *Data entry is time consuming, inefficient, difficult to navigate, and interferes with the doctor-patient relationship.*
- *Template-based notes degrade the quality of clinical documentation and care.* [14]

Impacts of Depersonalization on Quality of Care and Healing

The criticism of medicine as being too focused on the science of disease vs. the care of patients is not a new one. In a talk to medical students at Harvard Medical School in 1925, entitled The Care of the Patient, Dr. Francis Peabody had this to say:

> *The most common criticism made at present by older practitioners is that young graduates have been taught a great deal about the mechanism of disease but little about the practice of medicine—or to put it more bluntly, they are too 'scientific' and do not know how to take care of patients. . . For the secret of 'the care of the patient' is in caring for the patient.* [15]

A 1974 book by Dr. Mack Lipkin, *The Care of Patients*, brought us this insight:

> *Caring for the patient encompasses both the science and the art of medicine. The science of medicine embraces the entire stockpile of knowledge accumulated about man as a biologic entity. The art of medicine consists of the skillful application of this knowledge to a particular person for the maintenance of health or amelioration of disease. Thus the meeting place of the science of medicine and the art of medicine is in the patient. . . [and further] All experienced physicians know the great power of the reassurance they can give to patients who have faith in them.* [16]

The great problem today is the shortage of time for physicians to talk with patients, driven by the various factors we have seen in earlier chapters. Time has become money and health care is now just another commodity for sale in a marketplace driven by profits for corporate stakeholders, with most physicians working as employees under the thumbs of unseen managers. In a 2012 blog, I made this observation that becomes more true every day:

> *The missing element in today's depersonalized health care is time—listening and talking time between patients, their physicians and other health care professionals—during which patients can relate their narratives that can be integrated into plans for their care. We already know that trust between physicians and patients built over years improves medical outcomes and enhances healing.* [17]

Adverse drug interactions give us a good measure of their impact on serious reactions and death given today's dysfunctional medical practice environment as described above. We know that the average number of prescription drugs taken by Americans increases as they grow older, especially those with multiple chronic conditions. According to the Center for Disease Control and Prevention and the National Council on Aging, 92 percent of people over age 65 have at least one chronic condition and 77 percent have at least two. Medication-related problems are estimated to be among the top five causes of death among seniors, and a major cause of confusion, depression, falls, disability, and loss of independence. [18] We also know that many are under the care of multiple physicians, who often do not communicate well together. It is therefore no surprise that more than 2.7 million Americans experience serious adverse reactions, with 128,000 deaths from improperly prescribed drugs each year, with 1.9 million requiring hospitalization. It is estimated that 30 adverse reactions occur for every one leading to hospitalization, accounting for about 81 million adverse drug reactions among 170 million Americans taking drugs. Most are medically minor, such as muscle aches, slower reactions, or sleepiness, but they can cause many falls and accidents. [19]

Multiple physicians in different specialties treating patients, especially the elderly, with different conditions, are responsible for many drug interaction problems, often through lack of knowledge of what other drugs the patient is taking or how they fit into the patient's overall care and needs. Too often, no physician is in charge of the whole patient.

The expanding use of telemedicine gives us another example of the hazards and harms of virtual visits with physicians who never see, examine, or talk with the patient. One might think that the diagnosis of skin problems could be clinically useful and safe. But that is far from the case. A recent study by researchers posing as patients with skin problems sought help from 16 online telemedicine companies. Important diagnoses, such as syphilis, herpes, and skin cancer, were frequently misdiagnosed, key questions were not asked, and some of the online physicians were not licensed to practice where the patients lived. [20]

What does this mean for even more complex medical decisions, especially in later years balancing quality of life vs. longevity of life without meaning? That question exposes an even bigger hole in our depersonalized, fragmented health care system without a sufficient primary care foundation.

Concluding Comment

The above trends have become so entrenched in our new health care "system" that they are now part of the culture. They are difficult to change without fundamental reform, especially changing how we finance health care. We have evolved to a time when much of health care involves strangers taking care of strangers, with the patient's larger story lost in the shuffle. Today's new (and worse) culture in medicine and health care is a threat to medicine as a profession (as we will revisit in Chapter 13) and other healing arts. We have a long way to go to re-establish the primacy of the person as the reason for health care.

This leads us to the next chapter—how the traditional ethic of service in medicine and health care has been largely replaced by a business "ethic" of maximizing financial returns in today's largely corporate-dominated marketplace.

Endnotes:

1. French, M. More doctors are a click away, but some say it's not a healthy trend. *The Seattle Times,* January 14, 2016.
2. Geyman, JP. *Breaking Point: How the Primary Care Crisis Endangers the Lives of Americans.* Friday Harbor, WA. *Copernicus Healthcare,* 2011, pp. 168-170.
3. Mathews, AW. Secrets of the system: Physician panel prescribes the fees paid by Medicare. *Wall Street Journal,* October 27, 2010: A1.
4. Dorner, SC, Jacobs, DC, Sommers, BD. Adequacy of outpatient specialty care access in marketplace plans under the Affordable Care Act. *JAMA* 314 (16): 1749, October 27, 2015.
5. Terhune, C. Obamacare enrollees hit snags at doctors' offices. *Los Angeles Times,* February 4, 2014.
6. Brown, T. Out of network, out of luck. *New York Times,* October 15, 2013.
7. Murphy, T. Retail clinics, apps change doctor-patient relationship. *Associated Press,* September 9, 2015.
8. Beck, M. How telemedicine is transforming health care. *Wall Street Journal,* June 27, 2016: B1.
9. Relman, A. On breaking one's neck. *The New York Review of Books,* February 6, 2014.
10. Eddy, DM. *Clinical Decision Making: From Theory to Practice. A Collection of Essays from JAMA.* Boston. *Jones and Bartlett Publishers,* 1996, p. 1.
11. Pellegrino, ED. The medical profession as a moral community. Bulletin. *Bull N Y Academy of Medicine* 66 (3): 222, 1990.

12. Jonsen, A. Opening remarks. Symposium on Commercialism in Medicine. Program in Medicine & Human Values. California Pacific Medical Center, San Francisco: *Cambridge Quarterly of Health Care*, spring 2007.

13. Abelson, R, Creswell, J, Palmer, G. Medicare bills rise as records turn electronic. *New York Times,* September 21, 2014.

14. Friedberg, MW, Chen, PG, Van Busum KR et al. RAND Health Research Report. *Factors Affecting Physician Professional Satisfaction and Their Implications for Patient Care, Health Systems, and Health Policy.* Santa Monica, CA. RAND Corporation, 2013. Htpp://www.rand.org/content/dam/rand/pubs/research_reports/RR400/RR439/RAND_pdf

15. Peabody, FW. The care of the patient. *JAMA* 88: 877-882, 1927.

16. Lipkin, M. *The Care of Patients*. New York. *Oxford University Press,* 1974, p. 163.

17. Geyman, JP. Personhood: casualty of modern medicine. *The Huffington Post*, December 5, 2012.

18. Administration on Aging, 2012. Center for Disease Control and Prevention, 2012. National Council on Aging, 2014.

19. Light, DW. New prescription drugs: A major health risk with few offsetting advantages. Harvard University. *Edmond J Safra Center for Ethics*, June 27, 2014.

20. Beck, M. Websites misdiagnose ailments. *Wall Street Journal*, May 16, 2016: A6.

CHAPTER 9

CHANGING ETHICS IN MEDICINE
AND HEALTH CARE

The medical profession had a long history of a service ethic before it underwent its transformation during the last 60 years. When I went through medical school and graduate training, money was not part of our daily discussion. Upon graduation from medical school, we each took an oath, such as the Hippocratic Oath and the Physician's Oath. It was all about learning the art and science of medicine and what was in the best interest of the patient.

This chapter has three goals: (1) to briefly describe the traditional service ethic in the medical profession; (2) to give the main reasons for the replacement of that ethic by a "business ethic" of corporatized health care; and (3) to ask what kind of ethic will prevail in 21st century health care in this country.

The Traditional Service Ethic in Medicine

There has been a common theme of beneficence running through earlier centuries in medicine that transcended culture, religion, and history. Dr. William Osler, the best-known physician and medical educator in the English-speaking world at the turn of the 20th century, expressed it this way:

> *As the practice of medicine is not a business and can never be one, the education of the heart—the moral side of the man—must keep pace with the education of the head . . . . The profession of medicine is distinguished from all others by its singular beneficence.* [1]

123

Despite these historical traditions, however, there has also been a long-standing tension among physicians between altruistic service to patients and entrepreneurial self-interest. Dr. Edmond Pellegrino, whom we met in the last chapter, identified this dilemma facing the medical profession as a choice between two opposing moral orders— "one based in the primacy of our ethical obligations to the sick, the other to the primacy of self-interest and the marketplace." [2]

In the oaths that physicians take, they profess, as members of the medical profession, their dedication to the welfare of those they serve, beyond their own self-interest. As such professionals, they have been accorded special status through their role as healers. Moreover, as an unwritten contract with society, they have been given more autonomy than most other professions, at least in the past.

Despite the long historical precedent for a service ethic in medicine, it is obvious how far we have strayed from it as we look across the new landscape of corporatized medical practice and health care.

Today's Prevailing "Business Ethic" in Health Care

Most physicians are honest, hardworking, and dedicated to the best interests of their patients, but feel trapped in a system over which they have little control. There are many fine examples of the best of medical professionalism throughout the system, especially in the public sector's safety net, such as in community health centers, the Indian Health Service, and other underserved urban and rural areas. But many physicians, employed as they are by employers bent on "efficiency" and "production," feel constrained and controlled by the business "ethic" of our corporatized health care system.

How did this ethical transformation happen? Three main reasons, all inter-related, seem to explain this huge change in ethics and values.

1. Corporate takeover of health care, with shift to "shareholder capitalism."

We saw in Chapters 1 and 2 how corporations have taken over so much of the medical-industrial complex—from hospitals and other facilities to the drug and medical device industries. Recent decades have also seen consolidation as corporations got bigger, including expanding hospital systems that now employ a large part of the physician workforce.

Less recognized is a major shift in corporate missions and ethics that has evolved since the 1960s in this country. As Steven Pearlstein describes in a 2014 essay, "Corporations well into the 1960s were broadly viewed as owing something in return to the community that provided them with special legal protection and the economic ecosystem in which they could grow and thrive." He then describes how maximizing shareholder value and returns has become the dominant norm of corporate behavior, including shorter time horizons for investors and CEOs, squeezing employees, avoiding taxes, leaving communities in the lurch, and incenting CEOs with stock options. As a result, Gallup polls have shown a long, slow decline in the public's trust and respect for corporations—today, only Congress and HMOs are lower. [3] An early 2017 Harris poll found that only 9 percent of U. S. consumers believe pharmaceutical and biotechnology companies put patients over profits, while only 16 percent of health insurers do. [4]

Nobel laureate Milton Friedman, the University of Chicago's guru of market capitalism, stated this view very clearly in 1967:

> *Few trends could so thoroughly undermine the very foundations of our free society as the acceptance of corporate officials of a social responsibility other than to make as much money for their shareholders as possible.* [5]

Physicians have been caught up in the corporatization of medicine, losing autonomy in the process. In the 1960s, less than 10 percent of physicians were employed by hospitals, which were dependent on them for their hospital admissions. Today, almost two-thirds of U.S. physicians are employed by others, most by expanding hospital systems. Hospitals hire physician groups to gain market share and to raise their revenues through greater control over physician practices. According to the American Hospital Association, the number of physicians on hospital payrolls has increased by one-third since 2000. [6]

2. Self-interest trumping service

Unfortunately, there are too many examples of physicians giving up their service heritage for their own gain, often with little regard for patients' welfare. Here are some examples that show how widespread the sell-out of many physicians has become.

Hospitals

Prime Healthcare Service Inc., with a cardiologist CEO, has become a large for-profit hospital chain with 32 hospitals in a dozen states. It has recently been charged by the Justice Department for systematically increasing its Medicare revenues by setting quotas for hospital admissions and pressuring emergency room physicians to admit patients to the hospital unnecessarily, including falsification of records intended to justify hospital stays. [7]

Physician-owned specialty hospitals have emerged over the last three decades as a means of evading laws prohibiting them from referring their patients to hospitals in which they are invested. They focus on well-reimbursed procedures, especially in cardiovascular disease and orthopedic surgery, and cherry pick well insured patients. While they claim to offer more efficiency and value to patients, maximizing revenue is an obvious goal, since physician owners can "triple dip" by receiving income from performing a procedure, sharing in a facility profit, and increasing the value of their investment in the business. [8]

Ambulatory surgery centers (ASCs)

There are more than 4,000 ASCs across the country, typically privately owned between hospitals and physicians, but sometimes entirely owned by physicians and investors. Conflicts of interest are pervasive, even to the point that a 2003 article in *Medical Economics* described ways in which physician investors might avoid anti-kickback regulations. [9]

Imaging centers

Physician owners of CT and other imaging centers order two to eight times as many imaging procedures as those who do not own such equipment, amounting to an estimated $40 billion worth of unnecessary imaging each year. [10]

Urologists' ownership of radiation facilities

Some urologists have integrated intensity-modulated radiation therapy (IMRT) into their office practices, thereby allowing them to get around federal bans against self-referral of their patients with prostate cancer and gain high reimbursements. IMRT has not been shown to have better outcomes than other forms of radiation therapy. It has been shown that these urologists more than doubled their use of IMRT after adding this treatment to their practices. [11]

Conflicts of interest with the drug industry

These are common within the medical profession, including acceptance of highly paid roles as "consultants" to drug companies, giving talks more oriented to marketing than unbiased science, participating as "experts" developing clinical practice guidelines for use of a particular drug that they represent, and undisclosed financial arrangements with drug companies. [11,12] A recent study found that the drug and medical device industries had paid about $3.5 billion to physicians in the last five months of 2013, including some who no longer were practicing medicine and were serving on corporate boards or writing software used in laser-surgery machines. [14]

Conflicts of interest with the medical device industry

Manufacturers of medical devices seek out physicians to use and promote their products as a big part of their marketing programs. By 2011, there were surgeon-owned implant companies in 20 states, involved in such areas as cardiac, hip, and knee surgery. Surgeon owners can "double dip" by using devices made by their companies.[15] Another widespread practice that has received little scrutiny is the involvement of device representatives, really sales reps for their products, actively involved in the operating room during surgery, typically without informed consent of patients. [16]

Conflicts of interest between academic medical centers (AMCs) and industry

These are widespread, in many cases influencing what research is undertaken, how it is conducted, and whether or how it is reported (negative results often go unreported). [17,18] Dr. Jerome Kassirer, former editor of *The New England Journal of Medicine* and author of the excellent book, *On the Take: How Medicine's Complicity with Big Business Can Endanger Your Health*, summarized the problem this way in 2005:

> *Not one powerful medical center has declared war on financial conflicts. None has outlawed faculty participation in speakers' bureaus, participation in consulting arrangements that are thinly veiled marketing efforts, or completely eliminated company-sponsored meals. Many set no limits on stock options or income from patent royalties. Most have no rules about how often their faculty members can be involved with for-profit entities. And the rules that most institutions do invoke are often enforced irregularly. Few institutions have turned their conflict-of-interest*

issues over to a regulative body that is independent of the parent institution, but that is exactly what they should do. [19]

By 2015, conflicts of interest between AMCs and industry in this country were still rampant, as shown by a recent study reporting that 41 percent of investor-owned health care firms have directors with academic medical affiliations involving average annual compensation for board participation of $193,000, plus average ownership of more than 50,000 shares of stock. [20]

Medicare fraud

This is on the increase and is estimated to account for about 10 percent of the Medicare budget, mostly involving false billings by physicians, nurses, pharmacy owners, and other health professionals. The biggest criminal healthcare fraud takedown in the history of the Department of Justice occurred in 2015—a total of 243 people were arrested and charged with stealing $712 million from Medicare. [21] In 2016, in a national sweep against health care fraud, some 300 health care professionals were arrested and charged for fraudulent billings to Medicare and Medicaid. [22]

Dr. David Lotto, a psychoanalytic psychohistorian, gives us this insight concerning the decline of medical professionalism in recent decades:

> *There are far too many health professionals among us who are willing to bend, contort, and turn inside out, our traditional professional values. Too many are willing to accommodate to the values of the corporate world where protecting the wealth of those who are paying you becomes part of your professional function. Making this kind of accommodation has its rewards: mainly financial security and a comfortable middle class lifestyle. But like all Faustian bargains, there is a steep price to pay. The*

problem is that in order to avoid anxiety and guilt we come to share the moral blind spots of our corporate culture. [23]

Marc Rodwin, professor at Suffolk University Law School and author of the 1993 book, *Medicine, Money, and Morals: Physicians' Conflicts of Interest*, summarizes the problem this way:

American society's failure to face physicians' conflicts of interest squarely has led to major distortions in the way medicine is practiced, compromised the loyalty of doctors to patients, and resulted in harm to individual patients, society, and the integrity of the medical profession. Today medicine, money, and morals are often in dangerous conflict. They need not be. Many of these conflicts can often be reduced or rendered harmless through social policies. Designing new policies and institutions that hold physicians accountable to patients will be difficult. Yet we should not shrink from the challenge. For the difficulties of the status quo are far worse. [24]

Such a departure from the ethics of the 1950s, when Dr. Jonas Salk, having developed the first effective vaccine for polio, with some support from the March of Dimes, answered Edward R. Murrow's question about who would own the patent this way:

The American people, I guess. Could you patent the sun? [25]

3. Failure of self-regulation by the profession

These are some of the ways that the medical profession has fallen far short of its responsibilities to uphold its professional standards:

- Failure to rein in, or speak effectively against physician-induced demand—physicians' roles in ordering up to one-third of health care services that are inappropriate, unnecessary, sometimes harmful and even contraindicated. [26]

- Unwillingness to acknowledge and attempt to deal with lower quality of care in areas of the country with higher reimbursement rates and excess capacity of specialists and technology, as compared to areas with less capacity. [27]

- Silence and lack of leadership concerning cost-benefit and cost-effectiveness of new products brought to market by industry, in many cases involving physicians' conflicts of interest with manufacturers of products that fall below rigorous scientific criteria for their use.

- Failure to place any constraints on the epidemic growth of physician ownership and investments in health care services, such as specialty hospitals and physical therapy centers, wherein overutilization and profiteering goes unchecked. [28,29]

- Physicians' participation as "hired guns" conducting clinical trials in for-profit commercial research networks, without connections with academic medical centers and often without rigorous standards and with conflicts of interest between investigators and sponsoring drug companies. [30]

- Conflicts of interest with drug manufacturers, as authors of meta-analyses and systematic reviews of the literature, whereby scientists have financial interests in the results of the reviews. [31]

Which Ethic Will Prevail in the 21st Century?

The ACA has contributed to the medical profession's loss of its moral compass. The ACA has introduced new ways to compensate physicians and hospitals, including pay-for-performance, accountable care organizations, and bundled payments. All are unproven, and already have been found to add more ways to game the system. We still don't have a good system of how to pay physicians. Perverse incentives remain the norm in a largely for-profit health care marketplace, as Drs. Himmelstein and Woolhandler conclude:

> *There are many bad ways to pay doctors, and no particularly good ones. Other nations have achieved better outcomes, lower costs and fairer compensation of physicians using a variety of methods: fee-for-service, capitation, and salary; none is clearly best. The common theme isn't mode of payment, but a universal system with regulations that restrain costs and minimize the opportunities for profit and the risk of loss. . . Payment reform should focus not on manipulating greed, but on dampening it. Then the real motivations for good doctoring—altruism, social duty, and the glow we feel when we help our patients—can flourish.* [32]

Concluding Comment

As we have seen, the medical profession and other parts of the health system have become enveloped in a new business "ethic" that maximizes profits and has largely replaced the traditional service ethic of medical practice and health care. This is a moral crisis that cannot be fixed within the status quo. Unfortunately, this crisis has deepened after the 2016 election cycle, which turned the White House and both chambers of Congress to Republican control. This is how Dr. Arthur Caplan, professor of bioethics at New York University's Langone Medical Center and author of *Moral Matters: Ethical Issues in Medicine and the Life Sciences*, sees our current situation:

Trump needs to appease the paleocons and religious right to get things done. This makes it likely that bioethics will be swept back into the culture wars of the Bush era—Abortion, Contraception, Sexuality, Embryo research, Gene engineering, Enhancement issues, Chimera formation, Gender reassignment. All are back on the table. Individual rights will dominate arguments favoring the public good. Public health ethics will become hugely contentious.[32]

We will return to the decline of the professionalism in medicine in Chapter 13 and discuss three basic alternatives in Part Three, only one of which has the potential to re-establish service as the orienting ethic in health care.

Endnotes:

1. Osler, W. *On the Educational Value of the Medical Society. In Aequanimitas. With Other Addresses to Medical Students, Nurses, and Practitioners of Medicine.* Third edition. Philadelphia, PA, *Blakiston Company*, 1932.
2. Pellegrino, ED. The medical profession as a moral community. *Bull N Y Acad Med* 66 (3): 221, 1990.
3. Pearlstein, S. When shareholder capitalism came to town. *The American Prospect*, March/April 2014, pp. 40-48.
4. The Harris Poll, January 17, 2017.
5. Friedman, M. *Capitalism and Freedom.* Chicago. *University of Chicago Press*, 1967.
6. Bavley, A. Doctors Inc.: Medicine goes corporate as more physicians join hospital payrolls. *Kansas City Star*, January 17, 2014.
7. Evans, M. Hospital chain's CEO faces suit. *Wall Street Journal*, August 1, 2016.
8. Kahn, CN. Intolerable risk, irreparable harm: The legacy of physician-owned hospitals. *Health Affairs (Millwood)* 25 (1): 130-133, 2006.

9. Luxenberg, S. Invest in a surgicenter? *Medical Economics*, December 5, 3003, pp. 60-65.

10. Bach, PB. Paying doctors to ignore patients. *New York Times,* July 24, 2008.

11. Mitchell, JM. Urologists' use of intensity-modulated radiation therapy for prostate cancer. *N Engl J Med* 369: 1629-1637, 2013.

12. Geyman, JP. *How Obamacare Is Unsustainable: Why We Need a Single-Payer Solution for All Americans.* Friday Harbor, WA. *Copernicus Healthcare*, 2015, p. 54.

13. Campbell, P, Colizza, K, Straus, S et al. Financial relationships between organizations that produce clinical practice guidelines and the biomedical industry: A cross-sectional study. *PLOS Medicine,* May 31, 2016.

14. Whalen, J, Walker, J, Rockoff, D. Payments reveal range of doctors' ties with industry. *Wall Street Journal*, October 2, 2014: B7.

15. Carreyrou, J, McGinty, T. Taking double cut, surgeons implant their own devices. *Wall Street Journal*, October 8, 2011: A1.

16. Boodman, SG. Medical device employees are often in the O. R. raising concerns about influence. *Kaiser Health News*, November 15, 2016.

17. Bekelman, JE, Li, Y, Gross, CP. Scope and impact of financial conflict of interest in biomedical research: A systematic review. *JAMA* 289: 454, 2003.

18. Steinbrook, R. Gag clauses in clinical-trial agreements. *N Engl J Med* 352: 2160-2162, 2005.

19. Kassirer, JP. *On the Take: How Medicine's Complicity with Big Business Can Endanger Your Health.* New York. *Oxford University Press*, 207, 2005.

20. Anderson, TS, Good, CB, Gellad, WF. Prevalence and compensation of academic leaders, professors, and trustees on publicly traded U.S. healthcare company boards of directors: cross sectional study. *British Medical Journal* 351: 4826, September 29, 2015.

21. Graham, DA. The true face of Medicare fraud. *The Atlantic*, June 19, 2015.

22. Associated Press. Feds charge 300 in nationwide health care fraud sweeps. *New York Times*, June 22, 2016.

23. Lotto, DL. The corporate takeover of the soul of healthcare. *J Psychohistory* 26 (2):603-609, 1998.

24. Rodwin, MA. *Medicine, Money & Morals: Physicians' Conflicts of Interest.* New York. *Oxford University Press*, 1993, p. 247.

25. Smith, J. *Patenting the Sun: Polio and the Salk Vaccine.* New York. *William Morrow*, 1990, p. 159.

26. Schuster, M, McGlynn, EA, Brook, RH. How good is the quality of health care in the United States? *Milbank Q* 76 (4): 517-563, 1998.

27. Fisher, ES, Wennberg, DE, Stukel, TA et al. The implications of regional variations in Medicare spending. Part 2: Health outcomes and satisfaction with care. *Ann Intern Med* 138 (4): 288-298, 2003.

28. Medicare Payment Advisory Commission. Report to the Congress: Physician-Owned Specialty Hospitals. Washington, D.C.: MedPAC, March 8, 2005.

29. Mitchell, JM, Sass, TR. Physician ownership of ancillary services: Indirect demand inducement or quality assurance? *J Health Econ* 14: 2631-2689, 1995.

30. Bodenheimer, T. Clinical investigators and the pharmaceutical industry. *N Engl J Med* 3342: 1539, 2002.

31. Harris, R. Reviews of medical studies may be tainted by funders' influence. *Northwest Public Radio NOW,* October 12, 2016

32. Himmelstein, DU, Woolhandler, S. Global amnesia: embracing fee-for-non-service—again. *J Gen Intern Med* 29 (5): 693-695, 2014.

33. Caplan, A. Bioethics faces a rocky but navigable road. *Bioethics Today*, November 9, 2016.

CHAPTER 10

RELIGION AND MEDICINE: A BAD FIT

The question of appropriate authority in clinical deci-
sion making is a question of power and politics—macro and
micro—but it is also a question of ethics, political theory,
and policy. . . Where is the appropriate balance between
state, federal, and local authority? It is a recurrent issue in
American history—manifested now in struggles over such
visible issues as abortion policy or Oregon's "right to die"
legislation or California's medical marijuana statutes. [1]

—Charles E. Rosenberg, professor of the history of
science and Ernest E. Monrad Professor in the Social
Sciences at Harvard University

As observed above, religious views have always been part
of medical decision making under some circumstances, and how
it may affect outcomes of care remains an important question for
clinicians. This chapter explores this subject with three goals: (1)
to briefly describe two personal experiences during medical school
(Chapter 14) and my Mount Shasta practice years (Chapter 15) that
sensitized me to the problem of dealing with religious dogma in
medical practice; (2) to discuss two controversial issues—women's
reproductive rights and Death with Dignity, and show how patient
outcomes can be adversely impacted by religious dogma; and (3) to
consider what is happening in today's politics concerning both of
these issues.

Some Early Personal Experiences

Halfway through medical school, my wife and I attended a weekend retreat where a Presbyterian medical missionary described his work in the Belgian Congo. He was a surgeon who trained native residents to perform a number of surgical procedures, even including removal of gall bladders. With many color slides, he showed how he would walk back and forth supervising six surgeries going on at the same time. He also blessed and tried to convert every patient just before they were put under anesthesia. This turned me off, seeming to me to be inappropriate imposition of religious power. The Presbyterian Medical Mission was the largest such organization in the world at the time. Any thought that I might have had of considering such work disappeared when I was informed by the Board that my religious beliefs (agnostic) were not welcomed.

Later, in the mid-1960s in Mount Shasta, I had another experience that put me face to face in dealing with religious dogma in an urgent situation.

> *I had taken care of a Jehovah's Witness couple for a couple of years when the wife came in pregnant and wanted me to take care of her through the pregnancy, her second. She was Rh negative and her husband was Rh positive. There had been no problem with Rh incompatibility with her first pregnancy. We discussed that potential problem, how we would monitor the baby's blood carefully after delivery, and how we might need to refer the baby for urgent treatment in a larger hospital setting depending on the results of the baby's blood tests. This was way before Rh immunoglobin and the Rhig preventive shot; exchange transfusion was the treatment of choice if the baby developed jaundice and hemolytic anemia, with the worst outcome*

being kernicterus, brain damage that can cause cerebral palsy, hearing loss, and intellectual disabilities.

The delivery went well, and we started to check the baby's blood frequently for bilirubin, which results from the breakdown of the baby's red blood cells (Rh positive from the father's genes) when attacked by the mother's Rh negative antibodies. The level requiring emergency transport at that time was 17 or 18 milligrams per deciliter. Serial tests came up to 10, then 13, and I called the father to the hospital to talk with him and his wife about the need to consider emergency transport. I had first called my pediatrics consultant in Redding, 65 miles to the south, but he was not prepared to do an exchange transfusion. His recommendation was a Sacramento hospital. I talked with both parents for a full hour, explaining the high risk of doing nothing, but they steadfastly refused the possibility of any blood transfusion, despite hearing about likely serious outcomes for the infant with kernicterus.

What was I to do? As a physician, I was responsible for both the mother and infant. I decided to do what, to me, was the right thing—transport the baby regardless of what the parents wanted—and now. Fortunately it was a good day, with air transport available. I had read earlier about what a physician did in New Jersey when confronted with a similar circumstance when caring for a child of a Jehovah's Witness family after trauma required blood transfusions for their child—he got a court order.

So I called the County Attorney in Yreka, but it was a Friday and he was on his way to San Francisco for a weekend meeting with his colleagues from Northern California. My next call was to the County Attorney in Eureka in Mendocino County. He hadn't left yet, but didn't have a ready response to my dilemma. He would check on it and get back. Now it was mid-afternoon, and I made my decision—call for air med-evac from Medford, Oregon, to Sacramento, landing at our local airport just a few miles south of Mount Shasta to pick up the infant. Our nurses made all this happen as our latest blood test reached 16, and the child was on the way to Sacramento as a call came back from Eureka that a court order was in process. The child received excellent care in Sacramento, though ironically, the bilirubin level stabilized at 18, then slowly dropped so that an exchange transfusion was not done. Needless to say, I lost that family for further care, but would have made the same decision again.

Two Major Controversies Involving Religion and Medical Practice:

Expansion of Catholic hospital systems is accelerating around the country, partly by acquiring non-Catholic hospitals. This trend is posing an increasing threat to access to care in two major areas—women's reproductive services and end-of-life care. Ethical and Religious Directives for Catholic Health Care Services (the ERDs) are being enforced by the bishops vigorously in many parts of the country, holding their employed physicians to strict adherence to the ERDs or loss of employment. In many instances, health professionals employed by Catholic hospitals cannot provide counseling or referrals based on religious grounds. Nuns for many years have been more permissive in these areas, but increasingly the bishops are dictating what services can be provided. [2]

1. Women's Reproductive Rights

These are some of the ERDs restricting common needs of women in their childbearing years:

- Catholic hospitals may not promote or condone contraceptive practices.

- Abortion (that is, the directly intended termination of pregnancy before viability or the directly intended destruction of a viable fetus) is never permitted.

- In case of extrauterine pregnancy, no intervention is morally licit which constitutes a direct abortion.

- Direct sterilization of either men or women, whether permanent or temporary, is not permitted in a Catholic health care institution.

- Prenatal diagnosis is not permitted when undertaken with the intention of aborting an unborn child with a serious defect.

- Heterologous fertilization (that is, any technique used to achieve conception by the use of gametes coming from at least one donor other than the spouses) is prohibited because it is contrary to the covenant of marriage, the unity of the spouses, and the dignity proper to parents and the child.

- The free and informed health care decision of the person. . . is to be followed so long as it does not contradict Catholic principles.

- Catholic health care services must . . . require adherence (to the Directives) within the institution as a condition for medical privileges and employment.

- Other ERDs prohibit abortion even in cases of rape or incest and in-vitro fertilization [3-5]

There may be some variation from one institution to another as to how these Directives are interpreted under specific circumstances. Often there are gray areas when health care professionals are unsure how the ERDs will be interpreted. But the proscription against abortion is inviolate in all Catholic institutions.

Ten of the 25 largest health systems in the U.S. are Catholic-sponsored, where health professionals are prohibited from providing health services or honoring patients' health care requests in these areas. Washington State has the highest proportion of acute care hospital beds in Catholic hospitals—45 percent—of any state in the country. [6]

The following cases in two parts of the country indicate how extreme and harmful strict adherence to the ERDs can be:

- *Sierra Vista is a rural community about 80 miles southeast of Tucson, AZ with one hospital serving a three-county area. The local hospital had been secular until purchased in 2010 by the Carondelet Health Network, a member of Catholic-sponsored hospitals. ERDs were to be followed at the time of transfer of ownership. Shortly thereafter, a woman presented to the Emergency Room 15-weeks pregnant with twins after miscarrying one of the twins at home. The remaining twin had a heart beat. The attending physician concluded that any attempt to continue the pregnancy would pose high risks of loss of the child as well as hemorrhaging and infection for the mother. As he and the staff were preparing to complete the miscarriage, a hospital administrator intervened and ordered the patient transferred to another hospital 80 miles away, where she did receive necessary care. The medical staff felt misled since they had previously been assured that they could provide appropriate care for miscarriages. [7]*

- *A woman 18 weeks along in her pregnancy came to Mercy Health Partners, a Catholic-sponsored hospital in Muskegon, Michigan, where it is the only hospital with two campuses in the community. Her water had broken at home and contractions had started. She was told that she had premature rupture of the membranes (PROM), that nothing could be done, and to go home. She was not informed that there was almost no chance that the fetus could survive and was not counseled about risks of non-treatment to herself. She returned to the hospital the following morning with painful contractions, bleeding and an elevated temperature. Her contractions were monitored and she was given Tylenol. She was again sent home after the temperature came down. Later that same night, she returned to the hospital again in severe distress. While the staff was preparing to send her home, she delivered a very premature son, who died within hours. She soon developed infection that had developed after her membranes ruptured. The American Civil Liberties Union (ACLU) has filed a lawsuit contending that "a young woman in a crisis situation was put at risk because religious directives were allowed to interfere with medical care. . . . Patients should not be forced to suffer because of a hospital's religious conviction."* [8]

A 2012 national study of about 1,200 obstetrician-gynecologists found that 52 percent of those who practiced in Catholic hospitals experienced conflicts with their institutions over religiously-based policies for patient care. Restrictions were common concerning best treatment of ectopic pregnancy. Some physicians, contractually bound as they were, found these restrictions unacceptable, especially in cases where patients were already losing a pregnancy and/or the mother's health was at risk. [9] As Dr. Debra Stulberg, assistant professor of family medicine at the University of Chicago and lead author of this study, said about women wanting a tubal ligation after having a Caesarian section in a Catholic hospital: " [the prohibition against sterilization] means she will have to go to a separate hospital and have a second surgery, complete with the further risk of another round of anesthesia. It's not medically good for a woman to have two surgeries when she could have had one." [10]

2. Death with Dignity and End-of-Life Care

There are now five states in the U.S. where physicians are permitted to prescribe life-ending drugs to patients with terminal illness who choose, under certain requirements, to voluntarily end their lives: Washington State, Oregon, Vermont, Montana, and most recently California in 2015. These laws have become known as Death with Dignity, which allow patients who are suffering from a terminal illness to self-administer the drugs that hasten the end of their lives. Each such patient must have met these criteria:

- must be an adult resident of a state legalizing this practice,
- must have been diagnosed with an incurable, irreversible, terminal disease that will lead to death within six months,
- must have undergone a psychological examination to confirm absence of mental illness, including depression,
- must have had a second physician's confirmation of eligibility, and must have asked for the medication a total of three times, twice verbally and once in writing. [11]

If an individual has a physician in a Catholic hospital or clinic, he or she will not have this option to choose Death with Dignity. This is what the ERDs require on this matter:

- Catholic healthcare institutions may never condone or participate in euthanasia or assisted suicide in any way. [Dying patients who request aid in hastening the event] should receive loving care, psychological and spiritual support, and appropriate remedies for pain and other symptoms so that they can live with dignity until the time of natural death.

- Patients experiencing suffering that cannot be alleviated should be helped to appreciate the Christian understanding of redemptive suffering.
- A Catholic health care institution will not honor an advance directive that is contrary to Catholic teaching.
- Physicians are required to ignore end-of-life directives if they conflict with Catholic doctrine (in the case of a patient in a persistent, vegetative coma, similar to Terry Schiavo, tube feeding is required).

This is what happened to a patient in 2014 in a hospice affiliated with Providence Health & Services, a large Catholic healthcare network in Washington State:

As a resident of Washington State, which had passed a Death with Dignity Act in 2006, he had a right to seek medical help to end his life because of terminal brain cancer with the potential to become extremely painful. But his physician and other medical professionals charged with his care declined to provide him with information about aid in dying or referrals to other places that might be able to help him. Eventually, he decided to solve the situation on his own. He climbed into a bathtub and shot himself with a gun. [12]

Here is an 87-year-old patient's experience with cancer who was initially referred to a hospice affiliated with Providence Hospital in Seattle:

From the very first interview both social workers and nurses tried to force me to sign up for a chaplain consultation. I said no politely, explaining that I was secular, and had had several years to prepare my thoughts for death,

> *and had my books and friends . . . They spent long sessions of conversation trying to get me to see a chaplain "just once." . . . As a secular person, I found religion and supernatural practices untrue and unwholesome. It never occurred to me to mention Death with Dignity, so that was not an issue. It is very unpleasant to have nice nurses and social workers seated facing you trying to force you to sign up with something you don't believe in. They came and did this even when they had to come in and sign the transfer to the hospice I am now in which offers a chaplain but immediately takes no for an answer.* [13]

Physicians in Catholic institutions can, and are, fired if they fail to follow the ERDs. That happened to an Oregon physician after a pharmacist reported an end-of-life prescription to the physician's office, which was passed along to the medical director and then to a priest, who fired him. [14]

The Catholic Medical Association in California advises Catholic physicians not to accept Physician Orders for Life Sustaining Treatment forms (POLST). This is an excerpt from these instructions:

> *Because of the inherent risks of POLST orders, doctors and staff should not use or recognize POLST forms, nor will they execute an advance directive that conflicts with Catholic moral teaching.* [15]

All this Catholic dogma is against the grain of changing medical practice across the country. POLST programs have been adopted or are in development in 43 states. They are revocable at any time. These forms ask patients, if and when they have no pulse and are not breathing, to choose whether or not they want CPR/attempted resuscitation or Do Not Resuscitate (DNR). If they have a pulse and are breathing, they are further asked to choose among:

- *Comfort measures only.* Use medication by any route, positioning, wound care and other measures to relieve pain and suffering. Use oxygen, oral suction and manual treatment of airway obstruction as needed for comfort. Patient prefers no hospital transfer: EMS contact medical control to determine if transport indicated to provide comfort.

- *Limited additional interventions.* Includes care described above. Use medical treatment, IV fluids and cardiac monitor as indicated. Do not use intubation or mechanical ventilation. May use less invasive airway support (e.g. CPAP, BiPAP). Transfer to hospital if indicated. Avoid intensive care if possible.

- *Full treatment.* Includes care described above. Use intubation, advanced airway interventions, mechanical ventilation, and cardioversion as indicated. Transfer to hospital if indicated. Includes intensive care. [16]

Dr. Stuart Farber, the late family physician and pioneering director of the University of Washington's Palliative Care service, died in 2015 of acute myelogenous leukemia, the same disease his wife had at the same time. Their caregiving worked both ways along their journey, as each one's aggressive chemotherapy treatment failed and entered a palliative care phase. Despite his terminal disease, he left these inspiring words as his legacy to us:

> *Knowing that I am mortal is a sacred knowledge that makes each moment an awesome gift filled with opportunity for love, joy, and peace. It has transformed how I live my life. If I know I am mortal, then what is important? Sharing love and joy within my relationships: with myself, my wife, my family, my grandchildren, my friends, my colleagues, and the community in this very moment we are living.* [17]

Today's Politics Involving Religion in Medical Practice

It is both remarkable and dysfunctional that medical practice has become so politicized over the last 60 years. Decisions by politicians, leading an uninformed electorate, prevent the use of effective medical interventions that end up harming patients and their families' lives, all in the name of their own religious beliefs imposed on others. Today, as represented by all 2016 presidential candidates of the Republican party, this is being done on the basis of conservatism and "religious liberty" under the Constitution. It has become a hallmark of most Republicans at the state and federal levels to oppose abortion clinics and defund Planned Parenthood.

There are many ironies involved in these issues, including Ronald Reagan's statement during the 1984 presidential campaign, made in a synagogue on Long Island, supporting the separation of church and state:

> *We in the United States, above all, must remember that lesson, for we were founded as a nation of openness to people of all beliefs. And so we must remain. Our very unity has been strengthened by our pluralism. We establish no religion in this country, we command no worship, we mandate no belief, nor will we ever. Church and state are, and must remain, separate. All are free to believe or not believe, all are free to practice a faith or not, and those who believe are free, and should be free, to speak of and act on their belief.* [18]

At the other extreme, the Hyde amendment has been a little-known budget rider in Congress, renewed in every federal spending bill since 1976, that bans any federal funding from covering abortion services. [19] Fast forward to today's politics at the national level.

As president-elect, Donald Trump was quick to tell us that Roe v. Wade will be overturned under his U. S. Supreme Court, or that "women will have to go to another state for abortion care." [20] In the early days of his presidency, he issued a global gag rule prohibiting international organizations from receiving U. S. family planning funding if they provide, counsel, refer or lobby for abortion services. [21] Vice President Pence has vowed his intention to work with Congress to end taxpayer funding of abortion and abortion providers. [22] Rep. Tom Price (R-GA), the newly appointed incoming head of the Department of Health and Human Services (DHHS), has twice co-sponsored federal legislation that would define fertilized eggs as legal persons, thereby outlawing abortion but also common methods of contraception. [23] Sen. Jeff Sessions (R-AL), Trump's appointee as Attorney General, has over his entire career been anti-choice, anti-women, and has voted for defunding of Planned Parenthood and against reauthorization of the Violence Against Women Act. All of these proposed policies are both anti-women and irrational. According to a recent report from the Guttmacher Institute, the U. S. abortion rate reached a historic low in 2014, largely due to improved access to improved birth control. [24]

At the state level, Republicans in Texas have closed most of the state's abortion clinics, and have recently ended Medicaid funding for Planned Parenthood. A Colorado Family Planning Initiative started in 2009 with support from the Susan Thompson Buffet Foundation was eliminated even after it achieved these remarkable outcomes for about 30,000 participants using long-acting reversible contraceptives (LARCs)—40 percent decline in teen births, 34 percent decline in teen abortions, and a saving of $5.85 in short-term Medicaid costs per dollar spent on the program. [25]

Sister Joan Chittister, O.S.B., sums up the hypocrisy in the "pro life" movement this way:

> *I do not believe that just because you're opposed to abortion, that that makes you pro-life. In fact, I think in many cases, your morality is deeply lacking if all you want is a child born but not a child fed, not a child educated, not a child housed. And why would I think that you don't? Because you don't want any tax money to go there. That's not pro-life. That's pro-birth. We need a much broader conversation on what the morality of pro-life is.* [26]

At the local level, right here on San Juan Island with our only hospital being the Catholic Peace Island Medical Center (PIMC), the issues of full access to necessary and legal women's reproductive services and Death with Dignity have been discussed on many occasions, without resolution so far. The hospital project was never brought to a public vote on our island where voters voted for Death with Dignity by a 75-25 margin and where the percentage of over-65 residents is almost twice that of other Washington State counties. Nevertheless, physicians at PIMC cannot refer patients to Compassion & Choices in order help them understand their options and become eligible for Death with Dignity if they so desire. Instead, as the bishops' ERDs require, their continued suffering with terminal disease is "redemptive."

Can we return to a time when physicians, within a confidential doctor-patient relationship, are able to make medical decisions in the best interests of patients and their families without intrusion from religious dogmas that restrict their access to legal, appropriate, and helpful medical interventions? That freedom would certainly be consistent with the separation of church and state as firmly en-grained in the U.S. Constitution and advocated by such founders as Thomas Jefferson and James Madison.

Endnotes:

1. Rosenberg, CE. Anticipated Consequences: Historians, History, and Health Policy. In History and Health Policy in the United States: Putting the Past Back In. Stevens, RA, Rosenberg, CE, Burns, LR (eds). New Brunswick, NJ. Rutgers *University Press*, 2006, p. 27.
2. Geyman, JP. Catholic hospital systems: A growing threat to access to reproductive services. *The Huffington Post*, May 11, 2014.
3. United States Conference of Catholic Bishops, Ethical and Religious Directives for Catholic Health Care Services (5tg ed, 2009, available here [hereinafter Directive(s)].
4. O'Brien, J. How the Bishops' Directives derail medical decisions at Catholic hospitals. Catholics for Choice, December 4, 2013.
5. Uttley, L, Reynertson, S, Kenny, L, and Melling, L. Miscarriage of Medicine: The Growth of Catholic Hospitals and the Threat to Reproductive Health Care. ACLU and Merger Watch December 2013.
6. Ibid # 2.
7. Cohn, J. Unholy alliance. *The New Republic*, February 22, 2012.
8. Hausman, JS. ACLU's abortion lawsuit claims Catholic policy barred care for Muskegon woman at Mercy Health Partners. *All Michigan,* December 2, 2013.
9. Stulberg, DB, Dude, AM, Dahlqluist, I et al. Obstetrician-gynecologists, religious institutions, and conflicts regarding patient care policies. *Am J Obstet Gyn* 207 (1); 73e 105, 2012.
10. Rovner, J. When religious rules and women's health collide. NPR. May 8, 2012.
11. Stewart, K. At Catholic hospitals, a 'right to life' but not a right to death. *The Nation,* October 6, 2015. Available at: http://.www.thenation.com/article/at-catholic-hospitals-a-right-to...
12. Ibid # 11.
13. Harrington, M. Personal communication by email of patient's experience while hospitalized at Providence Hospital in Seattle, WA.
14. Ibid # 11.
15. http://cathmed.org/assets/files/POLST_Paradigm_and_Form.pdf
16. Landro, L. Patients' wishes protected. *Wall Street Journal*, June 9, 2014: A3.
17. Farber, S. Living every minute. *Compassion & Choices Magazine*, Fall. 2015, p. 13.

18. Daily Kos member. Ronald Reagan on the separation of religion and state. I agree. Conservatives might not. *Daily Kos*, July 1, 2014.

19. Covert, B. Bernie Sanders calls for repealing the Hyde amendment. *Nation of Change*, January 24, 2016.

20. Trump on SCOTUS, Roe v. Wade, *CBS News*, November 13, 2016.

21. Adelman, L. In first executive actions since historic Women's March, Trump moves to restrict access to reproductive health care worldwide. *Planned Parenthood Federation of America*, January 23, 2017.

22. Hackman, M. Pence vows support at antiabortion rally. *Wall Street Journal, January 28-29, 2017.*

23. Robbins, R. Trump win could boost movement to confer 'personhood' on fertilized eggs. *STAT*. December 9, 2016.

24. Dreweke, J. Anti-choice Republicans likely to ignore key reason for abortion rate decline. *Guttmacher Institute*, January 17, 2017.

25. Pollitt, K. Magic-bullet birth control? *The Nation*. June 8, 2015, p. 10.

26. Salzillo, L. Catholic nun explains pro-life in a way that will stun many (especially Republican lawmakers). *Daily Kos*, July 30, 2015.

CHAPTER 11

GROWING GAP BETWEEN MEDICINE
AND PUBLIC HEALTH

Medicine and public health share common goals, especially concerning the promotion of health and prevention of disease and injury. But they focus on two different targets—the individual patient and family for medicine, and the community
and population for public health. Their two approaches are also
quite different. The medical model aims to identify high-risk individuals and provide them help through screening, counseling, and treatment of asymptomatic or symptomatic disease. The
public health model attempts to reduce disease in the population
in such ways as mass education campaigns, environmental protection, labeling of foods, and taxation of tobacco. [1] Both fields
are involved with the prevention of disease in one of two ways:

- *primary prevention*: preventing the occurrence of disease or injury, such as by immunizations against infectious diseases, and
- *secondary prevention:* early detection of a disease process and
  intervention to reverse or lessen the progression of disease, such
  as by the use of mammography to screen for breast cancer.[2]

Though the two professions have much in common in their
goals, they have not always collaborated as well as they might, and
there remains some confusion about their roles in U.S. health care.
This chapter has three goals: (1) to bring some historical perspective
to the evolution of these two fields; (2) to compare their two differ-

ent paradigms, how they may or may not work together, and how the two fields have diverged in recent decades; and (3) to discuss the need for a new balance in the medicine-public health relationship.

Some Historical Perspective

While medical practice dates back over some 2,500 years, public health has a much shorter history of little more than 200 years. The U.S. Public Health Service traces its beginnings to a law passed by Congress in 1798, *The Act for the Relief of Sick and Disabled Seamen*, which led to the creation of a network of marine hospitals along coastal and inland waterways. The intent was to protect against the spread of disease from sailors returning from foreign ports and maintaining the health of immigrants entering the country.[3]

Public health and medicine worked together during the 19th century and early years of the 20th century in the primary prevention of disease, especially in reducing the incidence of many infectious diseases through sanitation and related efforts. Public health measures, such as water purification and pasteurization of milk, were credited with the sharp decline of deaths from gastroenteritis and lowering infant mortality rates.[4] Public health was largely responsible for reducing the death rates for typhoid fever and tuberculosis between 1900 and 1940 by 97 percent and 77 percent, respectively.[5]

Medicine and public health began to diverge in the early 20th century as independent schools of public health were established around the country after 1916. They brought together such disciplines as sanitary engineering, nutrition, epidemiology and biostatistics to strengthen the education and science of public health. While these have been important contributions, they also led to a growing gap between medicine and public health as clinical medicine shifted its focus away from preventive medicine toward the treatment of acute disease of individuals.[6]

Early detection of chronic disease became a high priority for both medicine and public health after 1950. Most of the gains have been through public health's interventions, such as population-based efforts to reduce smoking and encouraging exercise and lower-fat diets. Periodic physical examinations and screening by physicians have been less effective than population-based measures. [7] The CDC has estimated that the 30-year extension of life expectancy that Americans received in the 20th century was largely attributable to these ten most important achievements by public health: vaccination, motor vehicle safety, safer workplaces, control of infectious diseases, decline in deaths from coronary disease and stroke, safer and healthier foods, healthier mothers and babies, family planning, fluoridation of drinking water, and recognition of tobacco use as a health hazard. [8]

An important article in the *American Journal of Public Health* in 2010 summarized a major change in the status of public health vis-a-vis medicine after World War II in this country:

> *Social, cultural, and institutional changes provide the backdrop to the waning authority of public health that began in the years after World War II. In the 1950s, the rise of medical authority went hand in hand with the ascendance of the hospital as the center of treatment and research. Power was consolidated in corporate interests and given force by a general cultural ethos of mass consumption and market-driven health care. In the 1970s, a powerful discourse of personal responsibility for health and disease placed blame on individuals and implicitly absolved corporations that marketed harmful products such as cigarettes and lead paint and polluted the nation's water and air.[9]*

Table 11.1 shows three major stages in the relations between public health and medicine over the last 100 years. [10]

TABLE 11.1

Stages of Relations Between Public Health and Medicine

Period	Public Health	Medicine
Pre 20th century era of infectious disease: Cooperation	Focus on prevention: sanitary engineering, environmental hygiene, quarantine	Focus on treatment: direct patient care within comprehensive framework
Early 20th century era of bacteriology: Professionalization	Establishment of targeted disease control; Rockefeller Foundation report creates science-based schools of public health	Establishment of the biomedical model of disease, Flexner Report leading to standard science-based medical education
Post World War II era of biomedical paradigm: Functional separation	Focus on behavioral risk factors, development of publicly funded medical safety net (Medicaid/Medicare)	Pursuit of biological mechanisms of heart disease, cancer, and stroke, success with pharmacology, diagnostics, therapeutic procedures

SOURCE: The Institute for the Future. Health and Health Care 2010: The Forecast, the Challenge (2nd Ed). San Francisco: Jossey-Bass, 2003:166.

Two Different but Complementary Paradigms

Admittedly, there is a paradigm gap between public health and medicine, with the difference in broad terms being care of the population vs. the individual patient, respectively. Both paradigms share similar goals, and they should be complementary instead of separate ventures, as they are often perceived and conducted. The differences in their paradigms are shown by Table 11.2, the three pillars of public health, clearly different from the medical model. [11]

TABLE 11.2

The Three Pillars of Public Health

Assessment

The diagnosis of community health status and needs through epidemiology, surveillance, research, and evaluation of information about disease, behavioral, biological, environmental, and socioeconomic factors.

Policy Development

Planning and priority setting, based on scientific knowledge and under the leadership of the governmental agency, for the development of comprehensive public health policies and decision making.

Assurance

The securing of universal access to a set of essential personal and community-wide health services through delegation, regulation, or direct public provision of services.

Evaluation

SOURCE: The Institute for the Future. Health and Health Care 2010: The Forecast, the Challenge (2nd Ed). San Francisco: Jossey-Bass, 2003:166.

Although many medical schools are located on the same health science campuses as schools of public health, there is often an uneasy tension and distance between the two professions, with little collaboration between them and disinterest among many physicians. That separation is to the detriment of patients, families and communities.

Physicians and other health professionals in the medical care establishment may think that they are making more of a difference, patient by patient, than public health is able to do, but ongoing research shows the opposite. As one example, age-adjusted mortality rates for coronary heart disease dropped by almost one-half between

1950 and 1987 due much more from smoking cessation and diet than to such medical advances as coronary care units and cardiac bypass surgery. [12,13]

Public health makes more difference than medical care, so it needs to be given higher priority and be better funded to permit it to address the nation's needs, whether at federal, state, or local levels. It tends to be taken for granted until major challenges come along when we again recognize, often too late, how much we need it. Consider these examples of the critical need for public health when these challenges occur.

- *Katrina, 2005.* Despite credible warnings in advance of the hurricane, communication and coordination between public and private relief efforts were poor. At least 154 patients died in hospitals or nursing homes, which were not completely evacuated until five days after the storm hit. [14] The entire area's health care system was devastated by the storm; it took seven months for New Orleans Charity Hospital, the only level 1 trauma center for the entire Gulf Coast region, to reopen its trauma center in a temporary location in a suburban hospital. Many practicing physicians left the area, leaving critical shortages in primary care, hospital, mental health, and long-term care services even seven months after the storm. [15]

- *Hepatitis C epidemic.* Hepatitis C has become a major epidemic affecting 3.2 million Americans. Untreated, it can lead to liver cancer. Gilead's new drug, Sovaldi, can be curative, but costs about $84,000 for a full course of treatment, unaffordable for most patients with Hepatitis C who have an average annual income of just $23,000. [16] Dr. Steffie Woolhandler, whom we met in earlier chapters, observes this problem: "We're spending more and more treating disease, but less and less to prevent it. We're breaking the bank paying for Hepatitis C and cancer drugs, while drug abuse prevention, needle exchange programs and anti-smoking campaigns are starved for funds." [17]

- *Flint, Michigan disaster, 2016.* This most recent disaster was actually caused by failure of government at several levels, and exposes the preventable toxicity, especially in children, in the aftermath of lead poisoning of a large population. Between 6,000 and 12,000 children have been poisoned by very high lead levels in tap water, and are facing such serious future effects as developmental delays, learning difficulties, irritability, sluggishness and fatigue. Dr. Marc Edwards, an engineering professor at Virginia Tech and expert on municipal water quality, was shocked by the degree of lead contamination and the authorities' inaction in the face of their knowledge of the contamination. As he said, "The extent to which they want to cover this up exposes a new level of arrogance and uncaring that I have never encountered." [18]

Despite its importance, recognition and support for public health has been declining for many years. Dr. Karen DeSalvo, acting assistant secretary of the Department of Health and Human Services, observes:

> *Public health infrastructure has a history of being there when necessary, but on the other hand increasingly being marginalized and under-funded year after year. We are starving the infrastructure. Even though 80 percent of people's health is influenced by what happens outside of doctors' offices and hospitals, about 97 percent of funding goes to pay for medical services.* [19]

This under-funding is short sighted and ironic, particularly in view of new challenges confronting the country, ranging from increased use of addictive e-cigarettes among the young, increasing maternal mortality in states cutting back Planned Parenthood (e.g. Texas), contamination of drinking water supplies, increasing need for drug prevention programs, arresting the spread of Hepatitis C infection, and growing prevalence of depression with rising suicide rates to decreasing primary care and mental illness care capacity.

Need for a New Balance in the Medicine-Public Health Partnership

Medicine and public health need to work together for maximal gain, each is not enough alone. Their skills and expertise are complementary and interdependent, but there continues to be a dysfunction between the two professions that stands in the way of progress. Dr. David Satcher, former U.S. Surgeon General, called for a new partnership between the two in 2002, which is yet to happen:

> *What we need is a unique partnership between public health and medicine. Medicine means treating individuals, one at a time. Public health means working with community institutions like schools and worksites to promote good health and prevent what illness we can. Physicians and other health care providers need to bring more public health into their offices by offering prescriptions to change lifestyles, cease smoking, and increase physical activity. Public health also worries about cultural competency and barriers to access to high-quality health care. These concerns need to be reflected in the offices of physicians as well. Public health informs health care and vice versa; it's a partnership. That partnership is what the universal system of the future will need in order to succeed.* [20]

For such a new partnership to be established, both professions have to be willing to change. These are some of the changes needed:[21]

For medicine:

1. Recognize the limits of the medical model and embrace the goals of population health.

2. Replace attitudes of competition and distrust toward public health with a spirit of collaboration and mutual interdependence.

3. Change medical education to add new emphasis on preventive medicine and public health.

4. Encourage larger numbers of physicians to pursue graduate training in public health.

5. Advocate for national policies that can assure universal access to preventive and necessary health care services, strengthen primary care and public health infrastructures, and work toward greater accountability of the health care system as a whole.

For public health:

1. Revitalize and expand its state agency workforce, which is plagued by high vacancy rates and high annual staff turnover rates.

2. Expand and revise its multidisciplinary educational programs, including new emphasis on cross-cultural education and approaches to reduce racial/ethnic disparities in health care. [22]

3. Improve communications across agencies, facilities and disciplines in the public and private sectors, and enhance the public health system's capacity to gather, process, and share information.

4. Build new alliances with employers, health care organizations, and community organizations to develop and promote community health education programs and conduct research into the effectiveness of health-related interventions. [23]

5. Strengthen surveillance activities, including building international networks of public health laboratories, increasing information sharing among national surveillance authorities, and joint training of public health personnel. [24]

Concluding Comment

Despite many years of the dysfunctional gulf between medicine and public health, there is little progress toward the new partnership that is so needed. Public health remains grossly under-funded, and today's politics threaten to keep it that way, even as the needs grow. We have persistent disparities in access and outcomes of care, adoption of health promoting behaviors and health-promoting environments across racial, ethnic, and socioeconomic groups. Market forces exacerbate these problems, such as the unhindered marketing of "junk" foods to children by the food industry that has led to marked increases in prevalence of obesity and diabetes in American children [25], and the threat of increasing privatization of Medicare and Medicaid if the Republicans maintain control over much of our health policy. We will need greater public awareness and political will to create a new partnership between medical practice and public health. These observations by researchers from Columbia University's Mailman School of Public Health give us useful guidance for the future of public health:

> *Understanding the potential for achieving progressive social change as it moves forward will require careful consideration of the industrial, structural, and intellectual forces that oppose radical reform and the identification of constituencies with which professionals can align to bring science to bear on the most pressing challenges of the day.*

. . . If a commandment emerges from history, it is one that all sectors of the field can heed: find ways to align with constituencies, lend our science and our knowledge, and create a base of power for progressive social change. [26]

Endnotes:

1. Peng, R. The goals of medicine and public health. In: Hanson, MJ, Callahan, D (eds). *The Goals of Medicine: The Forgotten Issue in Health Care Reform*. Washington, D.C.: *Georgetown University Press*, 1999: 174-176.

2. Bodenheimer, TS, Grumbach, K. *Understanding Health Policy: A Clinical Approach.* (2nd edition). Stamford, CT: *Appleton & Lange*, 1998: 167.

3. Commissioned Corps of the U.S. Public Health Service. America's health responders. History. http://www.usphs.gov/aboutus/history.aspx

4. McKinlay, JB, McKinlay, SM, Beaglehole, R. A review of the evidence concerning the impact of medical measures on recent mortality and morbidity in the United States. *Intl J Health Serv* 19: 181, 1989.

5. Winslow, CEA. Who killed Cock Robin? *Am J Public Health* 34: 658, 1944.

6. Ibid # 1.

7. Terris, M. Healthy lifestyles: The perspective of epidemiology. *J Public Health Policy* 13: 186, 1992.

8. The Institute for the Future. *Health and Health Care 2010: The Forecast*, the Challenge (2nd edition). San Francisco, *Jossey-Bass*, 2003: 167.

9. Fairchild, A, Rosner, D, Colgrove, J et al. The EXODUS of public health: What history can tell us about the future. *Amer J Public Health* 100 (1): 54-63, 2010.

10. Ibid # 8, p. 166.

11 Ibid # 8, p. 168

12. Stamler, J. The marked decline in coronary heart disease mortality rates in the United States, 1968-1981: Summary of findings and possible explanations. *Cardiology* (Karger-Basel) 72: 11, 1985.

13. Goldman, L, Cook, EF. The decline in ischemic heart disease mortality rates. *Ann Intern Med* 101: 825, 1984.

14. Rhode, D, McNeill, DG, Abelson, R et al. Vulnerable and doomed in the storm. *New York Times*, September 19, 2005: A1.

15. Rudowitz, R, Rowland, D, Shartzer, A. Health care in New Orleans before and after Hurricane Katrina. *Health Affairs Web Exclusive*, August 26, 2006.

16. Surowiecki, J. The Financial Page. Biotech's hard bargain. *The New Yorker*, April 28, 2014.

17. Himmelstein, DU, Woolhandler, S. Public health's falling share of U.S. health spending. *Amer J Public Health*, November 12, 2015.

18. Edwards, M. As quoted by Lazarus, O. In Flint, Michigan, a crisis over lead levels in tap water. *Public Radio International*, January 7, 2016.

19. DeSalvo, K. As quoted by O'Donnell, J, Ungar, L. Public health gets least money, but does most. *USA Today*, December 8, 2015.

20. Satcher, D. As quoted by Mullan, F. Interview. David Satcher takes stock. *Health Affairs (Millwood)* 21 (6): 161, 2002.

21. Geyman, JP. *The Corrosion of Medicine: Can the Profession Reclaim its Moral Legacy?* Monroe, ME. *Common Courage Press*, 2008, pp. 260-261.

22. Betancourt, JR, King, RK. Guest editorial. Unequal treatment: The Institute of Medicine Report and its public health implications. *Public Health Reports* 118: 287-292, 2003.

23. News and Notes. IOM: Overhaul of Government public health infrastructure, new partners needed. *Public Health Reports* 118: 118-119, 2003.

24. Frenk, J, Sepulveda, J, Gomez-Dantes, O et al. The new world order and international health. *Brit Med J* 314 (7091): 1404-1407, 1997.

25. Nestle, M. Food marketing and childhood obesity—a matter of policy. *N Engl J Med* 353 (24): 2527-2529, 2006.

26. Ibid # 9.

CHAPTER 12

MARGINALIZATION AND CRIMINALIZATION OF MENTAL ILLNESS

The present situation, whereby individuals with serious mental illnesses are being put into jails and prisons rather than hospitals, is a disgrace to American medicine and to common decency and fairness. If societies are judged by how they treat their most disabled members, our society will be judged harshly indeed. [1]

—E. Fuller Torrey, M.D., psychiatrist, schizophrenia
researcher, founder of the Treatment Advocacy Center,
and author of *Out of the Shadows: Confronting
America's Mental Illness Crisis*

The fields of psychiatry and mental illness have undergone huge changes over the last sixty years, some misguided as events have unfolded, some for the better and others for the worse. As medical students in the 1950s, we were exposed to Freudian psychiatry, heard about psychoanalysis, and wondered about seemingly subjective, "soft" criteria for mental illness. Then came drug therapy and theories about the biology of mental illnesses. Though we now have many new drug treatments for mental illness today, we don't really know whether or how the drugs work as we try to deal with an epidemic of mental illness under an umbrella of changing definitions of mental health and mental illness.

This chapter takes on three goals: (1) to bring some historical perspective to the shifting societal debate on how best to deal with mental illness; (2) to show ways by which mental illness has been marginalized in our health care system; and (3) to describe the extent to which the more serious mental illnesses have been criminalized.

Some Historical Perspective

The history of mental illness and mental health in this country is a complicated one with shifting public perceptions and changing definitions reflecting social attitudes with some admixture of science. Here are some historical benchmarks of an ongoing story.

Hospital confinement of the mentally ill

The era of state mental hospitals started in 1773 with the opening of the Eastern Lunatic Asylum in Williamsburg, Virginia, and was followed in 1816 by a second psychiatric hospital in Baltimore. That era would last about 150 years, with the growth of very large public mental hospitals across the country to house the seriously mentally ill under often grotesque conditions as human warehouses. The number of inpatients in these facilities rose from 41,000 in 1880 to 559,000 in 1955, a growth of 13-fold compared to a 3-fold increase in the U.S. population. [2]

Mental health policy by the federal government

State governments were responsible for most mental health policy until the passage of the National Mental Health Act of 1946 and the subsequent creation of the National Institute for Mental Health (NIMH) in 1948. Under the leadership of Robert H. Felix, the NIMH soon set about substituting a community-based policy for many public mental hospitals. [3] After ongoing disputes about what to do next, the Community Mental Health Centers Act was passed in 1963, establishing community mental health centers as the cornerstone of the new federal policy, but without links to state mental hospitals, which still had about half a million inpatients. The concept was that these centers could offer preventive and early diagnosis services that would reduce the incidence of mental disorders and make long-term hospitalization unnecessary. [4]

In his classic book mentioned previously, Dr. Fuller Torrey laments the shift of priorities and funding from serious *mental illness* to milder anxiety, social adjustment, and *mental health* problems. In his words:

> *The most flagrant example of this diversion of resources has been the diversion of mental health professionals. Federal and state governments have spent literally billions of public dollars to train psychiatrists, psychologists, psychiatric social workers, so that there would be enough to provide care for the mentally ill. Once trained, however, the vast majority of these professionals decided to provide psychotherapy and counseling to people with mental health problems rather than to treat people who were mentally ill. In effect, for the past 40 years, we have trained mental health professionals when we should have been training mental illness professionals.* [5]

Deinstitutionalization

As a result of these events, there were only about 54,000 inpatients in long-term state mental hospitals in the U.S. at the beginning of the 21st century. Hospital care has now become mostly limited to short-term admissions during florid episodes of serious mental illnesses when patients are believed to pose significant risk to themselves or others. [6] In 2006, David Mechanic, director of the Institute of Health, Health Care Policy, and Aging Research at Rutgers University, and Gerald Grob, professor emeritus of the history of medicine at the same institution, summarized the confused system of mental health in this way:

> *The mental health system since the 1970s has included a bewildering variety of institutions: short-term mental hospitals, state and federal long-term institutions, private psychiatric hospitals, nursing homes, residential care facilities, community mental-health centers, outpatient departments of hospitals, community care programs, community residential institutions with different designations in different states, client-run and self-help services, among others. This disarray and the lack of any unified structure of insurance coverage or service integration has forced many patients with serious mental health illnesses to survive in homeless shelters, on the streets, and even in jails and prisons.* [7]

Advent of psychoactive drugs and decline of psychotherapy

Thorazine (chlorpromazine), introduced in 1955, was the first effective antipsychotic drug. It received widespread use after the passage of Medicare and Medicaid in 1965. As other psychoactive drugs came along, the shift from hospital care to outpatient drug treatment led directly to deinstitutionalization, with the discharge of many psychiatric patients from mental hospitals (Figure 12.1). Drug therapy also led to a major change in psychiatric practice, replacing psychotherapy—talking therapy—for the treatment of the seriously mentally ill. A majority of psychiatrists preferred to care for those with less serious mental *health* problems, such as anxiety disorders, leaving a vacuum in the care of those with serious mental illnesses, such as schizophrenia and bipolar disorder. By 1997, here is how Dr. Fuller described the situation as a psychiatric *Titanic:*

> *Deinstitutionalization has helped to create the mental illness crisis by discharging people from public psychiatric hospitals without assuring they received the medication*

*and rehabilitation services necessary for them to live suc-
cessfully in the community. Deinstitutionalization further
exacerbated the situation because, once the public psychiatric beds had been closed, they were not available for
people who later became mentally ill, and this situation
continues to the present. Consequently, approximately 2.2
million severely mentally ill people do not receive any psychiatric treatment.* [8]

FIGURE 12.1

NUMBER OF INPATIENTS IN PUBLIC MENTAL HOSPITALS , 1950-1995

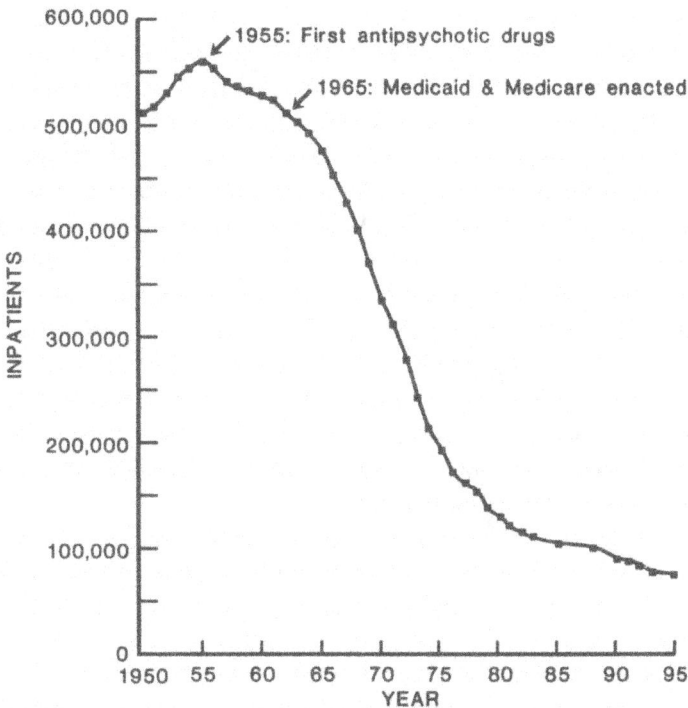

Source: Torrey, E. Fuller, *Out of the Shadows: Confronting America's Mental Illness Crisis*, New York, *John Wiley & Sons, Inc.*, 1997, p.9. Reprinted with permission.

The crisis in psychiatry

These are markers of how bad the psychiatric *Titanic* has become:

- The number of state psychiatric beds has dropped by 13 percent since 2010 to 37,679 beds; because of this shortage, many patients with severe mental illness are held in emergency rooms, hospitals, and jails ("psychiatric boarding"), without treatment as they await a bed, sometimes for weeks. [9]

- According to the 2016 annual report by Mental Health America on Americans with mental illness, more than one-half of them receive either insufficient treatment or none at all. [10]

- Access to urgent psychiatric care for children has become a crisis; a national shortage of child psychiatrists leads many suicidal children, those with bipolar disease and other serious mental illnesses to the ER, where care is inadequate and necessary follow-up care cannot be arranged. [11]

- Most psychiatrists have given up psychotherapy for brief "med check" visits [12]; many avoid care of the seriously mentally ill, instead setting up profitable practices caring for the "worried well," who are often seeking self-exploration therapy without a significant mental health problem. [13]

- The numbers of various mental health professions in practices not supervised by psychiatrists have grown markedly.

- Draconian cuts have been made in state budgets for mental illness and mental health care. [14]

- Psychiatric and behavioral problems among minority youth frequently result in school punishment or incarceration, but rarely mental health care. [15]

Revenue-producing markets

Fueled by the new emphasis on pharmacotherapy and the decline of time-intensive "talking therapy," the psychiatric profession was caught up with the shift toward revenue-producing services that we have seen in other parts of our system in earlier chapters. Drug companies lured psychiatrists to market their drugs in all kinds of ways, such as ongoing paid consultancies, speaking fees, and financing trips to conferences. Psychiatrists in private practice began making financial investments in private inpatient facilities to which they would admit their own patients, at which they may also be staff clinicians and have profit-sharing arrangements. [16] Diagnostic categories in psychiatry, always ambiguous and contested, became broadly expanded by medicalization of emotional and behavioral problems, with larger numbers of patients being labeled "disordered" in one way or another. Dr. E Haavi Morreim, associate professor of Human Values and Ethics at the University of Tennessee College of Medicine, summed up this transition in 1990:

> *The ongoing economic overhaul of medicine creates two basic imperatives—boosting profits and containing costs—that pose special   ethical and philosophical challenges for psychiatry. . . .The economic pressure to fill beds translates into a commensurate pressure on the profession to expand the concept of psychiatric illness, and with it the criteria for hospitalization and other extensive (revenue-producing) care. Moral problems arise at the clinical level when the psychiatrist is expected to apply such an expanded concept of illness to as many patients as possible.* [17]

Psychiatry was becoming a high-profit growth industry. Between 1970 and 1986, the proportion of proprietary inpatient psychiatric beds increased fifteen-fold as the number of free-standing psychiatric hospitals also saw dramatic growth. [18] When profits at general hospitals were declining, profit margins for psychiatric facilities were ranging up to 25 percent, or even as high as 30 percent for specialty services, such as adolescent units and eating disorder services. [19,20] Here are some benchmarks showing the extent to which the drive for profits has permeated the psychiatry profession:

- Among 4,000 attendees at the 2001 World Congress of Biological Psychiatry in Berlin, more than one-half were sponsored by drug companies, including business-class airfare and honoraria ranging from $2,000 to $10,000. [21]
- A joint venture between two of the country's largest for-profit behavioral health companies involving almost 400,000 Medicaid patients in Massachusetts kept receiving capitation dollars even after their systems of care collapsed; many children were left stranded in locked wards of psychiatric hospitals without arrangements for outpatient follow-up. [22]
- In 1998, Medicare expelled 80 mental health center programs after investigations found that 91 percent of claims were fraudulent. [23]

The growing epidemic of mental illness

Based on the numbers of Americans being treated for one or another mental health or mental illness conditions, we are in the midst of a raging epidemic in this country. The number of those disabled by mental disorders qualifying for Social Security Income (SSI) or Social Security Disability Insurance (SSDI) rose by almost two and a half times between 1987 and 2007, while mental illness has become the leading cause of disability in children. A large national survey by NIMH of randomly selected adults between 2001 and 2003 found that *46 percent* of those surveyed met criteria established by the American Psychiatric Association for having at least one mental illness! [24] While the pharmaceutical industry likes and promotes these numbers, voices of concern are being raised about this situation. Here are two examples:

- Dr. Daniel Carlat, psychiatrist practicing in a Boston suburb and author of the 2010 book, *Unhinged: The Trouble with Psychiatry—A Doctor's Revelations about a Profession in Crisis*, casts doubt on the chemical imbalance theory of mental illness, a key driver of drug therapy, calling it a myth. As he says, "It now seems beyond question that the traditional account of depression as a chemical imbalance in the brain is simply wrong."[25]

- Robert Whitaker, award-winning medical journalist and author of the 2002 book, *Mad in America: Bad Science, Bad Medicine, and the Enduring Mistreatment of the Mentally Ill*, states: "Prior to treatment, patients diagnosed with schizophrenia, depression, and other psychiatric disorders do not suffer from any known 'chemical imbalance.' However, once a person is put on a psychiatric medication, which, in one manner or another, throws a wrench into the usual mechanics of a neuronal pathway, his or her brain begins to function . . . abnormally." [26]

Marginalization of Mental Illness

Dr. Harold J Bursztajn, associate clinical professor of psychiatry at Harvard Medical School, describes mental health care in the U.S. today in these terms:

> *The major problem in the U.S. is that mental-health care tends to be marginalized—it's seen much more as a luxury than a necessity. The reimbursement system causes many institutions to prefer to provide high-tech and highly reimbursable medical care rather than the labor-inten-*

sive, poorly reimbursed mental-health services that are needed. There is also a misperception that mental-health care means simply prescribing medications that promise a quick fix. [27]

Here are some of the ways that mental health and illness care are marginalized in our society:

Stigma of mental disorders

This has been a long-standing problem, with many patients worried that admission of having a mental health disorder will adversely affect their jobs or social acceptance.

Lack of mental health parity

For many years, mental health care has not been accorded parity with physical illness by payers. Although federal legislation in 1996 and 2008 was intended to redress this problem, mental health benefits remain a second-class benefit by insurers, as this patient's story illustrates:

> *Michael Kamins, a marketing professor at the State University of New York, Stony Brook, was enraged when he opened a letter from his health insurer to find that it was no longer necessary for his 20-year-old son with bipolar disorder to see his psychiatrist twice a week. His son had recently been hospitalized twice and rescued from the brink of suicide, but the insurer would now pay for just two visits a month. His son later became violent and was re-hospitalized eight months later. His father is suing the insurer, OptumHealth Behavioral Solutions, which denies that it left the patient with insufficient care.* [28]

As this case demonstrates, insurers often invoke the lack of "medical necessity" in denying coverage of mental health disorders. They also disallow private coverage for a majority of people with severe mental illness, as shown in Figure 12.2. Even Medicare provides less coverage for mental health services, covering only 50 percent of their costs compared to 80 percent for other services. The Affordable Care Act attempted to improve this situation by specifying that mental health and substance abuse services are an essential health benefit, but many plans are exempt from this provision and Medicaid coverage is optional in many states. [29]

FIGURE 12.2

MENTALLY ILL PUSHED OUT OF PRIVATE COVERAGE

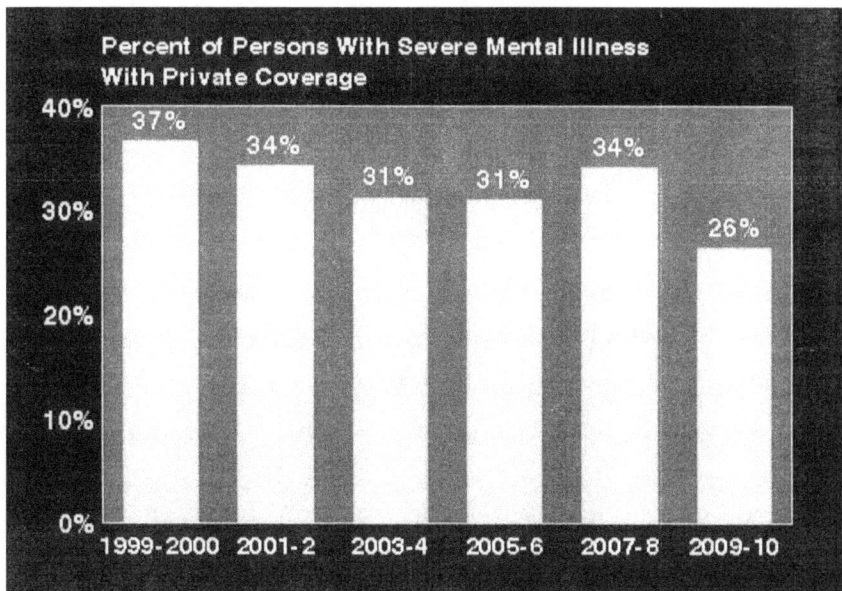

Percent of Persons With Severe Mental Illness With Private Coverage

Year	Percent
1999-2000	37%
2001-2	34%
2003-4	31%
2005-6	31%
2007-8	34%
2009-10	26%

Source: *Health Affairs* 2013;32:1723. Reprinted with permission

Limited access to psychiatric care

There is a national shortage of mental health professionals that limits access to care. A 2013 report by the U.S. Department of Health and Human Services found that 55 percent of the nation's 3,100 counties have no psychiatrists, psychologists or social workers as a result of budget cuts and retirements from the profession. [30] A 2013 study found that only 55 percent of psychiatrists would accept Medicare patients, with just 43 percent accepting patients on Medicaid. [31] A 2011 study in Boston found that only 12 percent of 64 facilities listed by Blue Cross Blue Shield of Massachusetts's PPO plan offered appointments even after being seen in an emergency room for depression and instructed to get a follow-up appointment within two weeks. [32] According to the American Psychiatric Association, 86 percent of psychiatrists listed in the Washington, D.C. exchange in 2016 were either unreachable or not taking new patients. [33]

Criminalization of Mental Illness

Two hundred years ago, the most common "treatment" for the seriously mentally ill was jail. Today, we have returned to that unacceptable and inhumane situation, largely because of the failure of the public mental health system. For many jailed patients, their only crime is their mental illness. Many are held without criminal charges because no other facilities are available. Others are charged with trivial "crimes", such as disorderly conduct. A small minority are charged with serious crimes, most often because their mental illness has been untreated. More than one-fifth of jails have no access to mental health services of any kind. After release from jail, only one-third of patients receive initial outpatient treatment and another one-third return to the streets, often later returning to jail. [34]

Jails have become today's asylums for the mentally ill after so many state mental institutions were closed in the 1970s. The largest mental health "treatment" facilities in the country are the largest jail systems—Cook County in Chicago, Los Angeles County, and New York City—where more than 11,000 prisoners are held on any given day. By comparison, the three largest state-run mental health hospitals have a combined 4,000 beds. [35] According to a 2014 report from the Treatment Advocacy Center, jails house ten times more mentally ill people than state mental hospitals, but many states have laws making it difficult or impossible to administer treatment over a prisoner's objections. [36]

A national survey of county jails in 39 states in 2016 found that three of four were seeing more seriously mentally ill inmates compared to five or ten years ago, that their staffs were ill equipped to care for these patients, and that only 42 percent of the jails offered psychiatric medications to them. Dr. Azza AbuDagga, lead author of the Public Citizen's Health Research Group's study, summarized the problem this way:

This growing problem is not solely a criminal justice problem. At its heart is evidence of the unacceptable failure of our public mental health system. [37]

Privacy concerns pose a major barrier to mentally ill persons receiving the best care in both their interest and the public interest. The current system discourages patients from seeking care because of the stigma of mental illness, and confidentiality is important to those who do seek care. In many states, we cannot require treatment of the mentally ill unless they are a danger to themselves or others, but there are limited requirements, varying by state, for health care providers to issue a warning if a patient is deemed dangerous. (Figure 12.3) [38]

FIGURE 12.3

LIMITED REQUIREMENTS TO DISCLOSE CONCERNS

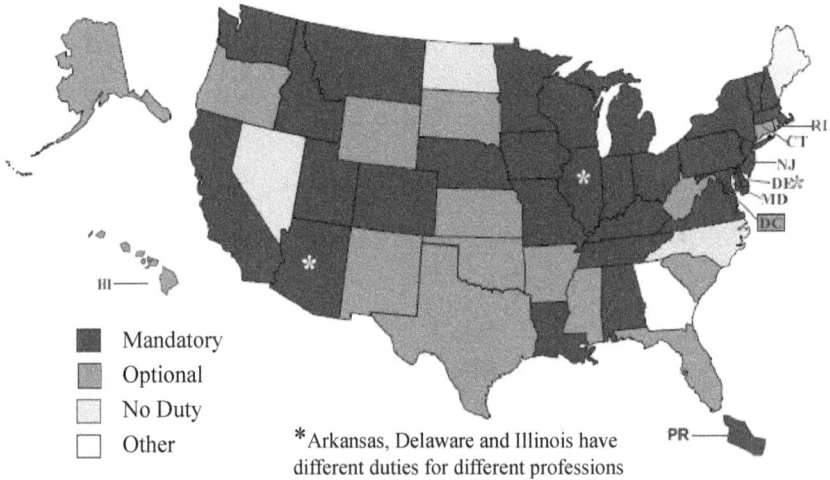

Mandatory
Optional
No Duty
Other

*Arkansas, Delaware and Illinois have different duties for different professions

Source: National Conference of State Legislators

This tragic story of a mass shooting in 2014 illustrates the barriers to appropriate management of the seriously mentally ill:

> *Three weeks before 22-year-old Elliot Rodger's murderous rampage near Santa Barbara, California, the sometime college student was questioned by sheriff's deputies outside his apartment. They were responding to a family member's concern about him. His mother was aware that her son had been posting bizarre videos on You Tube, but the deputies were unaware of them or that he had been in psychiatric care for years. For the deputies, this was a 'welfare check.' When questioned, he appeared to be calm, courteous, and not a threat to anyone. He did have guns stashed away in his apartment, about which his family was unaware, together with a blueprint to 'exact revenge on*

my enemies.' But the police would not have been able to search his apartment without a search warrant, and no evidence had been given them to get one. Three weeks later, at Isla Vista near the University of California Santa Barbara campus, he killed six people, wounded 14 others, and then apparently took his own life. [39]

Without sufficient information, there is no way for the police to assess the risk to the public when the family or others concerned do not share this kind of information with the police. As in this case, many mentally ill people can "hold it together" enough to appear "normal." Likewise, those with such information may often fear retribution from the mentally ill person. Moreover, federal privacy laws often thwart efforts by families to get critical information about a sick family member from health professionals. Like most other states, California's laws cannot involuntarily hold people in a mental facility for 72 hours' observation without having evidence that they are a danger to themselves or others.

The Treatment Advocacy Center tells us that about one-half of all individuals with severe mental illness are unaware of their illness and resist or reject treatment. That problem is called "anosognosia" or lack of insight. According to the NIMH, those with mental illness in treatment are 15 times less likely to engage in an act of violence than those not in treatment. Forty five states have adopted court-supervised treatment programs, known in different states as *assisted outpatient treatment (AOT)* or *mandatory outpatient treatment*, for patients who do not voluntarily comply with necessary medical and psychiatric care. [40] Research in New York State has found that 81 percent of those so treated were able to get and stay well, and that 90 percent were more likely to keep appointments and stay on medication. AOT has also been found to reduce rates of imprisonment, homelessness, emergency room care, and annual Medicaid costs. [41]

Concluding Comment

It is clear that the above that the fields of psychiatry and mental illness are at a more primitive level than we should expect despite all of the supposed advances of drug therapy in recent decades. There really is an epidemic of mental illness in this country, which needs to be given higher priority, including changes in laws that should require evaluation and treatment in an effort to prevent mass killings and other criminal activity. We need more science in the treatments that are used for the mentally ill, tighter oversight by the FDA, and less chance for the pharmaceutical industry to market drugs that are ineffective, including their off-label use. As with medical care, we also need fundamental restructuring of our way of financing health care, that shifts from market profit-taking to a public service ethic, as will be discussed further in Part Three.

Endnotes:

1. Torrey, EF. Severely mentally ill more likely to be in jails than hospitals, report shows. Public Citizen's Health Research Group. *Health Letter* 26 (6): 3, 2010.

2. Torrey, EF. *Out of the Shadows: Confronting America's Mental Illness Crisis.* New York. *John Wiley & Sons, Inc,* 1997, pp. 81-82.

3. Felix, RH, Bowers, RV. Mental hygiene and socio-environmental factors. *Milbank Memorial Fund Quarterly* 26: 125-147, 1948.

4. Grob, GN. *From Asylum to Community: Mental health policy in Modern America.* Princeton. *Princeton University Press,* 1991.

5. Ibid # 2, p. 185.

6. Mechanic, D, Grob, GN. Rhetoric, realities, and the plight of the mentally ill in America. In Stevens, RA, Rosenberg, CE, Burns, LR. (eds) *History & Health Policy in the United States: Putting the Past Back In.* New Brunswick, NJ. *Rutgers University Press*, 2006, p. 229.

7. Ibid # 6, p. 239.

8. Ibid # 2, p. 10.

9. Ollove, M. Amid shortage of psychiatric beds, mentally ill face long waits for treatment. *Pew Charitable Trusts,* August 2, 2016.

10. Nutt, AE. Report: More than half of mentally ill U.S. adults get no treatment. *The Washington Post*, October 19, 2016.

11. Luthra, S. Scarcity of mental health care means patients—especially kids—land in ER. *Kaiser Health News*, October 17, 2016.

12. Harris, G. Talk doesn't pay, so psychiatry turns instead to drug therapy. *New York Times*, March 5, 2011.

13. Dembosky, A. Psychotherapists gravitate toward those who can pay. *Kaiser Health News*, July 15, 2016.

14. Lacy, M, Sack, K, Sulzberger, AG. States' budget crises cut deeply into financing for mental health programs. *New York Times*, January 21, 2011.

15. Marrast, L, Himmelstein, DU, Woolhandler, S. Racial and ethnic disparities in mental health care for children and young adults: A national study. *Intl J Health Services,* August 12, 2016.

16. Weithorn, LA. Mental hospitalization of troublesome youth: An analysis of skyrocketing admission rates. *Stanford Law Review* 40: 773-838, 1988.

17. Morreim, EH. The new economics of medicine: Special challenges for psychiatry. *The Journal of Medicine and Philosophy* 15: 97-98, 1990.

18. Dorwart, RA, Schlesinger, M. Privatization of psychiatric services. *Amer J Psychiatry* 145: 543-553, 1988.

19. Gopelrud, EN. Effects of proprietary management in general hospital psychiatric units. *Hospital and Community Psychiatry* 37: 832-836, 1986.

20. Shahoda, R. Specialty services boost psych providers. *Hospitals* 60: 56-62, 1986.

21. Torrey, EF. The going rate on shrinks: Big PhRMA and the buying of psychiatry. *American Prospect,* July 15, 2002, p. 26.

22. Wolfe, SM. Unhealthy partnership: How Massachusetts and its managed care contractor shortchange troubled children. Public Citizen Health Research Group. *Health Letter*, 17 (2): 1, 2001.

23. Wrich, J. *Brief summary of audit findings of managed behavioral health services.* Chicago. J Wrich & Associates, 1998.

24. Angell, M. The crazy state of psychiatry. *New York Review of Books*, 2012.

25. Carlat, D. As quoted by Marcia Angell, Ibid # 18.

26. Whitaker, R. As quoted by Marcia Angell, Ibid # 18.

27. Bursztajn, HJ. Interview by Louis Jacobson. *Princeton Alumni Weekly*, February 6, 2013.

28. Gold, J. Advocates say mental health 'parity' law is not fulfilling its promise. *Kaiser Health News,* August 3, 2015.

29. Rowan, K, McAlpine, DD, Blewett, LA. Access and cost barriers to mental health care by insurance coverage, 1999-2010. *Health Affairs* (10): 1723-1730, 2013.

30. Fields, G, Dooren, JC. For the mentally ill, finding treatment grows harder. *Wall Street Journal*, December 21, 2013: A1.

31. Pear, R. Fewer psychiatrists seen taking health insurance. *New York Times*, December 11, 2013.

32. Boyd, JW, Linsenmeyer, A, Woolhandler, S et al. The crisis in mental health care: A preliminary study of access to psychiatric care in Boston. *Ann Emerg Med* 58 (2): 218-219, 2011.

33. News release. American Psychiatric Association, May 16, 2016.

34. Wolfe, SM. Criminalizing the seriously mentally ill: Two decades later. Public Citizen's Health Research Group. *Health Letter* 27 (7), July 2011.

35. Fields, G, Phillips, EE. The new asylums: Jails swell with mentally ill. *Wall Street Journal*, September 26, 2013: A1.

36. Capsules. Report: Jails house 10 times more mentally ill than state hospitals. *KHN Blog,* April 8, 2014.

37. Bradbery, A, Goodwin, D. National survey shows county jails unequipped, over-whelmed with seriously mentally ill inmates. *Public Citizen News*, September/October 2016, p. 4.

38. Fields, G. Families of violent patients: 'We're locked out' of care. *Wall Street Journal*, June 8-9, 2013: A 1.

39. Blood, MR, Abdollah, T. California rampage shows gaps in mental health law. *Associated Press*, May 28, 2014.

40. Assisted outpatient treatment—frequently asked questions. Treatment Advocacy Center, 2013. Available at: htpp://www.treatmentadvocacycenter.org/component/content/arti…

41. Murphy, T. Mass shootings and a mental-health disgrace. Op-Ed, *Wall Street Journal*, October 9, 2015: A 13.

CHAPTER 13

DECLINE OF PHYSICIANS'
PROFESSIONALISM AND AUTONOMY

A major power shift has occurred for physicians over the last 60 years in health care. Although physicians played a dominant role in shaping the directions and content of health care up to the 1960s, they now have to dance to the tune of insurers, hospital systems, managed care plans, employers, and to a lesser extent, the government through its public programs. As we saw in Chapter 9, physicians largely fell right in line with all these corporate changes, lacking the cohesion and organizational power to resist them. Some were lured to pursue their own self-interest over the needs of patients in the evolving market-based system.

This chapter has two goals: (1) to discuss the decline of professionalism in medicine; and (2) to describe the major reasons for and impacts of losses in physicians' clinical autonomy.

Decline of Professionalism

As a takeoff point for discussing these issues, it is useful to look at widely accepted characteristics of professions and professionals, as listed in Table 13.1. [1] Note especially the emphasis on public service above personal reward and professionals' obligations to set ethical criteria and discipline unprofessional conduct.

We discussed in Chapter 9 the many ways whereby many physicians in recent decades have put their own self-interest above the public interest, as well as the extent to which the medical profession

TABLE 13.1

Characteristics of Professions and Professionals

A profession possesses a discrete body of knowledge and skills over which its members have exclusive control.

The work based on this knowledge is controlled and organized by professional associations that are independent of both state and capital (i.e., the marketplace).

The mandate of these associations is formalized by a variety of written documents, including laws covering licensure and regulations granting authority.

Professional associations are the ultimate authorities on the personal, social, economic, cultural, and political affairs relating to their domains, and they are expected to influence public policy and inform the public within their areas of expertise.

Admission to professions requires prolonged education and training; the professions are responsible for determining the qualifications and (usually) the numbers to be admitted, the substance of training, and the requirements of its completion.

Within the constraints of the law, the professions control admission to practice and the terms, conditions, and goals of the practice.

The professions are responsible for the ethical and technical criteria by which their members are evaluated, and have the exclusive right and duty to discipline unprofessional conduct.

Individual members remain autonomous in their workplaces within the limits of rules and standards laid down by the associations and relevant laws.

Professionals are expected to gain their livelihoods by providing service to the public in the areas of their expertise.

Members are expected to value performance above reward.

Professions and professionals must be moral and are held to higher standards of behavior than are non-professionals.

Professionalism is an ideal to be pursued.

Source: Cruess, R, Cruess, S, Johnston, S. Renewing professionalism: An opportunity for medicine. *Acad Med* 74: 878-884, 1999.

has failed to regulate itself. Lack of willingness to see Medicaid patients, despite its expansion under the Affordable Care Act (ACA), is one glaring example of the profession's failure to serve the public today. Overall, 30 percent of office-based U.S. physicians will not accept new Medicaid patients today, while the percentages of non-acceptance are higher in some specialties—40 percent in orthopedic surgery, 44 percent in general internal medicine, and 56 percent in psychiatry. There are many reasons for this, of course, including gross under-reimbursement rates and administrative complexities, but this contributes to major barriers to Medicaid patients' access to care. Dr. Lawrence P. Casalino, Livingston Farrand Professor in the Department of Healthcare Policy and Research at Weill Cornell Medical College, brings us this insight:

> *We live in an era in which, for better or worse, market-based solutions are dominant and policymakers tend to view physicians as self-interested actors. Little or no attention is paid to physician professionalism or to the possible effects of policies on professionalism. Policies that are based on this view may be justifiable if many physicians are indeed seeking to maximize their incomes and refusing to accept even a slight reduction in income as the price for helping to provide care to the most vulnerable patients in our society. A 5% commitment campaign would be a meaningful, highly visible demonstration of physician professionalism—of putting patients first.* [2]

Dr. Lawrence Hergott, cardiologist and professor of medicine at the University of Colorado School of Medicine, notes that:

185

> *"External forces" are weighing down upon the profession. These forces are imposed by interests largely driven by economics and profit. [This process] is the "devolution of medicine."* [3]

As a result of the above trends, the public's trust in physicians and medical leaders in this country has dropped markedly over the last 50 years. In 1966, almost three-quarters of Americans had great confidence in the leaders of the medical profession; that number has fallen to about one-third, with only 23 percent expressing a great deal or quite a lot of confidence in the U.S. health care system. A 29-country survey conducted between 2011 and 2013 found that the U.S. ranks near the bottom of trust levels. The researchers concluded that: "If the medical profession and its leaders cannot raise the level of public trust, they're likely to find that many policy decisions affecting patient care will be made by others, without consideration of their perspective." [4]

Most of organized medicine, through the AMA and specialty organizations, has been ineffective in restoring a leadership role of the medical profession in the direction of health care. This is not to say, however, that the profession has not made some attempts to reverse the above trends in an effort to restore its professional and moral standing. One good example is the *Charter on Medical Professionalism* that was developed in 2002 by the ABIM Foundation, the ACP-ASIM Foundation, and The European Federation of Internal Medicine. It identified the three core principles that should underpin medical professionalism—primacy of patient welfare, patient autonomy, and social justice. (Table 13.2) [5]

Another important effort to rebuild the public trust in medicine was taken by the Institute of Medicine in 2011 (now the National Academy of Medicine) with its report, *Clinical Practice Guidelines*

TABLE 13.2

Fundamental Principles for Medical Professionalism

Principle of primacy of patient welfare. This principle is based on a dedication to serving the interest of the patient. Altruism contributes to the trust that is central to the physician-patient relationship. Market forces, societal pressures, and administrative exigencies must not compromise this principle.

Principle of patient autonomy. Physicians must have respect for patient autonomy. Physicians must be honest with their patients and empower them to make informed decisions about their treatment. Patients' decisions about their care must be paramount, as long as those decisions are in keeping with ethical practice and do not lead to demands for inappropriate care.

Principle of social justice. The medical profession must promote justice in the health care system, including the fair distribution of health care resources. Physicians should work actively to eliminate discrimination in health care, whether based on race, gender, socioeconomic status, ethnicity, religion, or any other social category.

SOURCE: Project of the ABIM Foundation. ACP-ASIM Foundation and European Federation of Internal Medicine. Medical professionalism in the new millennium: A physician charter. *Ann Intern Med* 136(3):244, 2002.

We Can Trust, which set a higher bar to avoid conflicts of interest for experts convened to set these guidelines. [6] Some medical organizations have led the way toward health care reform in the public interest, including Physicians for a National Health Program (PNHP) and the American Public Health Association. Leaders in other medical societies, such as the American Society of Clinical Oncology (ASCO), have called upon their organization to embrace reform in their cancer patients' best interests. Drs. Ray E. Drasga and Lawrence H. Einhorn appealed to their colleagues in these words in 2014:

> *With the ACA now the law of the land, and its reten-*
> *tion of the private insurance industry at the center of the*
> *health system, the trend toward high-deductible health*
> *plans, underinsurance, and cost shifting to patients will al-*
> *most certainly worsen. Fifty-nine years of private-sector*
> *solutions have failed. There needs to be a major paradigm*
> *shift in our approach to funding health care in the United*
> *States. Because ACA will fail to remedy the problems of*
> *the uninsured, the underinsured, rising costs, and growing*
> *corporate control over caregiving, we cannot in good con-*
> *science stand by and remain silent. Life is short, especially*
> *for some patients with cancer; they need help now.* [7]

The traditional social contract of the medical profession with society has been broken, raising the question of what will happen next? Can medicine renew its social contract with society? Drs. Julius Richmond and Leon Eisenberg of Harvard Medical School called for this effort in 2000:

> *The medical profession needs to re-establish its social*
> *contract with society. It must stop viewing public officials*
> *as the enemy and develop better ways of responding more*
> *broadly to the interests of the public.* [8]

Drs. Pellegrino and Relman urged a much more proactive role of medical associations at about the same time:

> *Today, the dominant influence on professional asso-*
> *ciations is economic, and the tension between self-interest*
> *and ethical principles is greater than ever. This conflict is*
> *eroding the moral foundations of all professional associa-*
> *tions, not only in medicine, but in law, education, and even*
> *the ministry.*

Physicians must now choose more definitively than ever whether their professional associations will assert the primacy of ethical commitment or shed any pretense of being moral enterprises and instead, allow economic considerations to dominate their policies.[9]

Decreasing Clinical Autonomy

How different from the 1960s, when you could open your own office, recruit your own staff, choose your consultants in all of the specialties based on their competence and caring for patients, be in charge of your own schedule, and take time for house calls, from which you learned so much about the patient, his/her family and circumstances relating to health care. In his recent book, *Doctored: The Disillusionment of an American Physician*, Dr. Sandeep Jauhar, a cardiologist, reminds us that house calls accounted for about 40 percent of doctor-patient encounters before World War II, compared to less than 1 percent today. [10]

The ACA has been a disaster for physicians in solo or small group practice. They must choose between two payment tracks for Medicare reimbursement—one whereby their performance exceeds "quality" benchmarks could lead to potential bonuses, the other being to become part of larger systems, such as accountable care organizations, where the pressure is to reduce costs and restrict care. Small practices confront increasing bureaucracy and overhead to meet the ACA's reporting requirements (the latest proposed payment regulations took up 962 pages in April of 2016). [11,12] Small practices caring for patients with socio-economic determinants that lower outcomes of care are also disadvantaged since "quality" measures are predictably lower than for more affluent patients.

Today, many physicians in independent private practice are finding it too difficult and costly to continue practice, faced as they are with increasing overhead, a growing bureaucracy concerning records and billing, and the volatility of the insurance market, rendered more complex and volatile by the ACA's changing requirements. [13] Under these circumstances, beyond the control of physicians, solo and small group practice have virtually disappeared. Physicians have been leaving independent practice in droves, relieving themselves of the hassles and costs of a small business and attracted by more secure and predictable incomes, fixed hours, guaranteed vacation, a 401 (k), health insurance, and medical liability coverage. [14]

Most physicians today are employed by others, especially by large hospital systems. According to the AMA, about 60 percent of family physicians and pediatricians are employed by hospitals, as well as 50 percent of surgeons and 25 percent of surgical subspecialists. This change inevitably leads to higher prices and revenues to hospitals acquiring physician groups. [15]

As hospital employees, physicians are salaried under contract and are pressured by administrators to be maximally "productive," meaning ordering up as many tests and procedures needed to meet their employers' (and sometimes shareholders') revenue goals. As we saw in Chapter 5, the impact on primary care has been severe, as illustrated by Timothy Hoff's observation from his 2010 book, *Practice Under Pressure: Primary Care Physicians and Their Medicine in the Twenty-First Century.* [16] (page 67 of Chapter 5)

Employed physicians are increasingly being treated like cattle without much say in how they practice medicine, as illustrated by these pressures imposed upon them by their employers:

- They don't get away from increased paper work, as their continued administrative burdens include time-consuming data entry into EHRs, dealing with the greatly expanded International Classification of Diseases (ICD-10) coding system of diagnostic codes (expanded from 14,000 to 70,000 in its latest version), and trying to resist pressures by their employers to "upcode" for maximal reimbursement by payers. [17] A 2014 study found that family physicians and internists were spending more than 17 percent of their time on administrative tasks, exceeded only by psychiatrists at 20 percent. [18] According to the 2016 Medscape Physician Compensation Report, more than one-half of U. S. physicians spend more than 10 hours per week on paperwork.[19]

- They have to deal with misleading "quality" measures under value-based payment systems, such as pay-for-performance (P4P), which many physicians find frustrating and of doubtful clinical value. [20]

- They are increasingly being tracked by hospital administrative staff to measure how well they are meeting institutional goals, such as the average number of days per hospital stay of adults; some physicians worry that this approach may lead to pressures to avoid older and sicker patients. [21]

As a result of these trends, the doctor-patient relationship has been compromised in a number of ways, including shorter visits with less face-to-face time with patients, and greater use of the computer during visits. Some insurers are intruding upon physicians' efforts to integrate care of their patients, as revealed by a recent report of private Medicaid managed care plans in Iowa cutting off patients' access to the Mayo mothership just across the border in Rochester, Minnesota, from their Mayo-affiliated primary care clinics in Iowa.[22]

Based on all these changes, it is no surprise that physicians' satisfaction with their practices has been dropping with burnout rates and early retirements increasing. The 2015 Medscape Physician Lifestyle Report found that almost one-half of respondents to a large national study had burnout, as defined by loss of enthusiasm for work, feelings of cynicism, and a low sense of personal accomplishment. Burnout rates for family physicians and general internists increased from 43 percent to 50 percent between 2013 and 2015, with the most common complaint being "too many bureaucratic tasks." [23] In another response to these pressures, some physicians are opting for concierge practice, setting up their own independent practices for a limited number of patients who pay an annual retainer fee for a broad range of services whenever needed. As one such physician said: "Unless you remain independent, you will have no say in what kind of medicine you practice." [24]

Concluding Comment

If professionalism can be restored, where will the forces come from? Efforts to do so within the profession have been inadequate. The public lacks awareness, cohesion, organization, and political power to do so, and society has still not demanded answers to two fundamental unanswered questions—Who is the health care system for? and Should health care be a public service or a for-profit business enterprise? History has shown that the medical profession and other health profession organizations have lacked the power (and concerted motivation) to counter the corporate business ethic.

Rosemary Stevens, professor of history and sociology of sciences at the University of Pennsylvania and arguably the leading medical historian of our times, asks these questions of the medical profession:

> *What is the future of medicine in the public sphere, as expressed through its professional organizations? Will the profession continue to be just one of many competing interest groups, whose influence will continue to wane? Or is there a basis on which the professional organizations of medicine might assume a new position of moral leadership in American health care?* [25]

Endnotes:

1. Cruess, R, Cruess, S, Johnston, S. Renewing professionalism: An opportunity for medicine. *Acad Med* 74: 878-884, 1999.

2. Casalino, LP. Professionalism and caring for Medicaid patients—the 5% commitment. *N Engl J Med* 369: 1775-1777, November 7, 2013.

3. Hergott, L. As quoted by Coates, AD. Colorado cardiologist sounds 'the eternal Yes!'. WAMC Northeast Public Radio, July 26, 2013.

4. Blendon, RJ, Benson, JM, Here, JO. Public trust in physicians—U.S. medicine in international perspective. *N Engl J Med*, October 23, 2014.

5. Project of the ABIM Foundation, ACP-ASIM Foundation, and European Federation of Internal Medicine. Medical professionalism in the new millennium: A physician charter. *Ann Intern Med* 136 (3): 243-246, 2002.

6. Greenfield, S. Rebuilding trust in medicine: How the public can interpret differing guidelines. *Health Affairs Blog*, November 17, 2015.

7. Drasga, RE, Einhorn, LH. Why oncologists should support single-payer national health insurance. *Journal of Oncology Practice*, January 17, 2014.

8. Richmond, JB, Eisenberg, L. Correspondence. Medical professionalism in society. *N Engl J Med* 342 (17): 1288, 2000.

9. Pellegrino, ED, Relman, AS. Professional medical associations: Ethical and practical guidelines. *JAMA* 282 (10): 984, 1999.

10. Jauhar, S. Bring back house calls. *New York Times.* Op-Ed, October 15, 2015: A31.

11. Woolhandler, S, Gaffney, A, Himmelstein, DU. Slow medicine: Assessing the ACA in the political fog. *MedPage Today*, August 26, 2016.

12. Findlay, S. Doctors raise concerns for small practices in Medicare's new payment system. *Kaiser Health News*, August 25, 2016.

13. Keegan, DW, Woodcock, E. Insurance exchanges: 6 crucial questions for physicians, October 15, 2013. www.medscape.com

14. Smith, Y. The stealthy, ugly growth of corporatized medicine. Op-Ed, *Naked Capitalism*, April 29, 2014.

15. Rosenthal, E. Apprehensive, many doctors shift to jobs with salaries. *New York Times*, February 13, 2014.

16. Hoff, T. *Practice Under Pressure: Primary Care Physicians and Their Medicine in the Twenty-First Century.* Piscataway, NJ. *Rutgers University Press*, 2010, pp. 16-17.

17. Doctors' paperwork increasing, 2012-2013. Physician Compensation Report. *Medscape.*

18. Woolhandler, S, Himmelstein, DU. Administrative work consumes one-sixth of U.S. physicians' working hours and lowers their career satisfaction. *Intl J Health Services* 44 (4): 635-642, 2014.

19. Sinsky, C, Colligan, L, Li, L et al. Allocation of physician time in ambulatory practice: A time and motion study in 4 specialties. *Ann Intern Med* online, September 6, 2016.

20. Ryan, J, Doty, MM, Hamel, L et al. Primary care providers' views of recent trends in health care delivery and payment. *The Commonwealth Fund and the Kaiser Family Foundation*, August 5, 2015.

21. Mathews, AW. Hospitals prescribe big data to track doctors at work. *Wall Street Journal*, July 11, 2013: A1.

22. Leys, T. Mayo rebuffs Iowa Medicaid managed-care contracts. *The Des Moines Register*, March 24, 2016.

23. Peckham, C. Physician burnout: It just keeps getting worse. *Medscape*, January 26, 2015.

24. Rao, A. Doctors transform how they practice medicine. *Kaiser Health News*, May 15, 2013.

25. Stevens, RA. Public roles for medicine in the United States: Beyond theories of decline and fall. *Millbank Q* 79 (3): 327, 2001.

PART TWO

THEN AND NOW:
A PERSONAL PERSPECTIVE,
1956 to 2016

CHAPTER 14

MEDICAL EDUCATION

Many physicians wanted to become a doctor from childhood. That was not me. Although my father was a radiologist, medicine was the last thing I wanted to consider as a kid, for two small reasons. First, at age seven, I was trotted off with my two sisters to the hospital for a tonsillectomy, as was in vogue at the time for minimal indications, like just being a kid. I never forgot that ether anesthesia, and kept well away from the ether smells around hospitals for some years to come. Another minor but formative incident was fainting dead away to the floor, while taking another person's pulse in a first-aid course when about 13. That led me to question whether I could ever deal with blood and other things medical.

On entering Princeton University in 1948, my first decision was to join the Navy ROTC program, with the goal of becoming a Navy pilot after graduation. I was not a fast enough reader at the time to consider the humanities or a social science major (that problem disappeared years later when doing editorial work). I settled for a major in Geology—interesting enough until hitting courses in physical chemistry and crystallography. I had no idea what I would do after graduation in 1952, except to first serve out my three years of active duty in the Navy. Having flunked the eye test, however, because of too much astigmatism even having never worn glasses, I didn't go to Pensacola for flight training, but to a destroyer in the Pacific.

It was on one of those long days at sea when I came upon an excellent book, *The Human Body*, by Dr. Logan Clendening from the

University of Minnesota. That was really interesting. I would pick it up between bridge watches and read on. Why had I not considered medicine? That could combine my interest in people with science that was directly relevant to serving people.

Pre-Med

After being processed out of the Navy at Treasure Island in the Bay Area, I enrolled at the University of California Berkeley to complete my pre-medical requirements. That was almost all of them, with just one chemistry course from Princeton counting. I also soon realized that I would have to get straight A's in all of these courses, which would take a year and two summers. The problem was how my Princeton grades translated to the UC system. I was at the bottom of the top-third of my class, which I found later converted to a number below the threshold for an interview at UCLA medical school.

Fortunately, with all A's a year later, I was accepted at Washington University in St. Louis, as well as the University of California San Francisco medical school (UCSF) after two good interviews. Having grown up in California and dating my soon-to-be wife, Gene, another Californian, that decision was clear—enroll at UCSF.

The Medical School Experience

Gene and I got married during the summer before the start of medical school and settled into a small apartment near the UC Berkeley campus, as she completed her student teaching year there.

Medical school classes were smaller in those days, with few women. Our Class of 1960 had just 84 students, with seven women. The first year of the curriculum was still on the Berkeley campus because the initial basic science building was demolished on the San Francisco campus in the fire and earthquake of 1906. Ours was the last class to take the first year in Berkeley, as it finally was relocated to the San Francisco campus a year later.

After our first year in Berkeley, Gene and I moved to an apartment just ten blocks from the UCSF campus. We were a close-knit class, less than one-third the size of today's UCSF medical school classes. A few of us were a bit older, having recently completed our military obligations. The curriculum then was sharply divided between the first two basic science years and the last two clinical years, with very few electives. The basic science courses were mostly taught by lectures, without much small group teaching. We had almost no direct contact with patients until the last two years, when the clinical clerkships started in the various specialties, mostly hospital based. It was in these years that I first heard frequent disparaging comments by some faculty about the LMDs, local general practitioners, "up country." That has always annoyed me as an example of unnecessary, and often ill-informed, town-gown attitudes.

Although medical technology had advanced considerably since World War II, the overriding emphasis during our medical school experience was more on service and care for the patient—to take personal responsibility for your patients. There was a strong emphasis on history taking, learning each patient's story as the main way to make a diagnosis. A physical examination would follow, with laboratory testing much more limited than today. Our physical diagnosis training was at Laguna Honda Hospital, an institution in the almshouse tradition from the Middle Ages dedicated to the care of all patients without regard to their financial assets—where the philosophy of care was that "the body is a garden to be tended rather than a machine to be fixed", as Dr. Victoria Sweet describes in her excellent book, *God's Hotel: A Doctor, A Hospital, and a Pilgrimage to the Heart of Medicine.* [1]

I liked everything in medical school, from internal medicine to surgery to psychiatry. I could see early on that I wanted to be involved in all of these areas in the care of the whole patient. I took two general practice preceptorships just to make sure, one in Santa Rosa, more of a suburban practice in Sonoma County, the other in Dunsmuir, a rural railroad town in Siskiyou County, with Dr. Bill Reynolds. The rural experience convinced me that I would head for broad-breadth general practice in a rural area where a physician could make a difference. Bill and I became close friends and later colleagues for many years.

The last year of medical school was exciting, as it is today, as soon-to-graduate seniors decide upon their choices for graduate training. General practice was not yet a specialty (it became so in 1969 with the formation of the American Board of Family Practice). Most of our class selected residencies in the traditional specialties, most commonly internal medicine or one of the surgical fields. Many faculty were disparaging about general practice. I heard more than a few times that "You're too smart to be a GP."

Only seven in our class wanted to become generalists, and we had to figure out how best to prepare ourselves for a broad-breadth practice for patients of all ages. Most future general practitioners first took a rotating internship, with rotations through all of the major specialties. A few then went into practice, but most took more training, sometimes in general surgery, some combination with internal medicine, or in general practice residencies. I applied to big county hospitals for rotating internships, was admitted to Los Angeles County General Hospital (LA County) the next year, with plans for an additional two-year GP residency to follow.

UCSF is one of U.S. medical schools that carries on a long tradition, the Gold Headed Cane, established by the Royal College of Physicians in England in the 17th Century as a symbol of art, culture, and achievement in medical practice. [2] I was surprised and honored to be selected by the faculty and my classmates for this honor as our Class of 1960 graduated.

Gene had been teaching primary grades through most of our medical school years, and our first son, Matt, was born in November of my senior year. Soon after graduation we were off to the Los Angeles area to get ready for the internship.

Graduate Training

L. A. County (The "Big House") had 3,500 beds in 1960, second in size only to Cook County Hospital in Chicago. It was, as it is today, a major teaching hospital, trauma center, and safety net institution for the large population of the county. There were multicolored stripes on the hallway floors helping to guide you to parts of the hospital. When a patient was brought into the Emergency Room, a blanket was put on him or her to designate urgency for care. A red blanket sent the patient directly up to surgery or intensive care, a maroon blanket required care within 20 minutes. The obstetrical service accounted for 13,000 deliveries a year. As an intern on that service (I did two months of OB), I could count on seven deliveries every 24-hour shift.

That was a great year. Interns had lots of responsibility. There was always a resident available when you needed help. Teaching rounds included faculty from the University of Southern California medical school, while some faculty were volunteering their time from community practice. That was where I first met Dr. Gabriel Smilkstein, a family physician in nearby Claremont, when rotating through the Jail Service, a general practice service on the hospital's 13th floor. He was an excellent teacher, was dedicated to community service, and became a colleague in later years at the University of California Davis.

You could encounter almost anything on the Jail service. I recall one day when, after pushing open the heavy barred door, I found a man on the floor, not breathing and turning blue. Of course that called for mouth-to-mouth breathing, CPR and so forth. He was resuscitated from his drug overdose of heroin, but then I would wonder for a while whether he had TB or not. Fortunately, my tuberculin test never did turn positive.

It was soon time to apply for a two-year general practice residency. There were a number of good ones at that time, mostly in county hospitals, including Ventura, San Bernardino, Alameda, and Santa Rosa in California, and in Denver, Colorado. Having spent time in Santa Rosa during my medical school preceptorship, I was familiar with the Sonoma County Hospital program. Since it was also close to Gene's family in Marin County, that decision was a no-brainer.

The GP residency at Sonoma County dated back to 1938. For most residents, it was a two-year program providing excellent training for practice in any setting, especially in rural areas. It has been for many years a "residents hospital." Patient care within its walls was provided by residents in consultation with community physicians in all specialties from the surrounding community. During my time there, 1961 to 1963, we had ten residents, five in each year, and with readily available consultants, we ran the hospital. Our residents' call system after hours and on weekends included one of us in the hospital for ER and acute problems on the wards, second on call for OB, and third on call for surgery or anesthesia.

Again, as at L.A. County, we residents had plenty of responsibility, but help was always available if needed. A good example was for fracture care. When we encountered a fracture that we could reduce and cast, we would call the attending orthopedist from town, describe the fracture and x-ray, and proceed, knowing that the orthopedics faculty would be regular attendees at our next teaching rounds when all of our cases would be presented and discussed.

The hospital then was a couple of miles out in the country from the town of some 35,000 (not true today since the area has grown so much). As a resident at night in an upstairs call room for the ER, we could hear the siren of the ambulance coming from miles out. Rushing down to the ER, we could encounter most anything. I recall one occasion when a gurney was brought in with a man who wouldn't talk. His blood pressure was 120/80, pulse 72 and regular, with good color. Bringing down the blanket over him revealed an elaborate handle of a knife embedded in his chest. He still wouldn't say anything as he was rushed up to surgery, where the knife was carefully removed, having just missed his heart. The back story later was that he was a Navy officer just back from the Language School in Monterey, had just killed his girl friend with that fancy knife obtained in Japan, and had intended to kill himself.

Our program had rotations through all the traditional specialties, with both inpatient services and outpatient clinics. Under close supervision, we learned procedural skills in surgery (including hernia repair, appendectomy, hysterectomy and cholecystectomy), obstetrics (including Caesarian sections), anesthesia, and closed reductions in orthopedics. As well, we gained experience in acute mental health problems through our 72-hour hold, locked psychiatric ward.

We residents also had the latitude to make changes in our teaching program. One such example during my time was to initiate an Allergy Clinic. We put together teaching materials, protocols for care, and invited allergists from the community as attending physicians. It was remarkable how many excellent clinicians and teachers would volunteer their time to get involved with the residency program, almost all on a voluntary basis.

In his book, *The Santa Rosa Reader,* Dr. Rick Flinders, a UCSF graduate and graduate of the residency in 1980, collated the four traditional pillars of this program, dating back some 65 years, in this way:

I. Supervised Autonomy: A model of teaching and learning in which residents experience the "heat" of primary responsibility—with supervision—for the care of patients.

II. An Environment of Academia: In which students teach and teachers learn.

III. A Tradition of Humanism and Social Justice: In which we acknowledge that access to care is the equal right of all patients, and that professional medical training is also an intense period of personal growth and development.

IV. A Strong Family Medicine Identity: That residents experience and identify with what it means to be a family physician. [3]

As we went through the program, we learned a lot from the resident group just a year ahead of us. We were also very interested in where they would go when they finished the program and how they would go about it. "Practice management" became an area we needed to know more about, and we toured the offices of some of the local family physicians to learn more about that. In most cases, graduates of the program would go out and start up their own practices, usually in a rural community in California or another western state, though some joined small group practices. Today, most medical graduates start their practice careers as employees of large hospital systems or another employer. In our day, we were all self-employed.

The long tradition of service and teaching at Sonoma County Hospital has endured to this day, as recounted in Dr. Flinder's book. Three name changes have occurred over these years—from Sonoma County Hospital to Community Hospital of Sonoma County to today's Sutter Medical Center of Santa Rosa. It is now owned and operated by Sutter Hospital based in Sacramento, which has continued its dedication to the residency program.

During the second residency year, Gene and I took an exploratory trip up through the Pacific Northwest looking for a place to settle and practice the next summer. Our priority was for a small community as a place to make a difference and raise our family. We stopped at Hood River, OR; Anacortes and Pullman, WA; Moscow, ID, Whitefish and Kalispell, MT. Of those, Kalispell appealed to us most at the time—beautiful country, west of the Divide, good hospital and schools, and a welcoming medical community. There was a small, unincorporated community a mile or two out of town on the Flathead River with no physician. So we drew up plans for a 1,000 square foot office and talked to a general contractor, who agreed to build the office on a lease-purchase basis over the winter and spring.

The contractor changed his mind during the winter, however, so all bets were off. Come June, as we completed the program, we didn't yet know where we would land. We headed north again, little knowing that we would be back in Santa Rosa six years later in another role, or that the Flathead River would flood the next year, which would have taken out our office had we gone ahead with our plans!

Endnotes:

1. Sweet, V. *God's Hotel: A Doctor, A Hospital, and a Pilgimage to the Heart of Medicine*. New York. *Riverhead Books*, 2012.
2. Macmichael, W. *The Gold-Headed Cane*. Springfield, IL. *Charles C. Thomas*, Seventh Edition, 1953.
3. Flinders, R. *The Santa Rosa Reader: A Personal Anthology from the Family Medicine Residency, 1968-2011*. Santa Rosa, CA. Sonoma County Medical Association, 2012.

CHAPTER 15

RURAL PRACTICE

My First Practice:
Mount Shasta, California, 1963-1969

First stop heading north was to visit our friend, Bill Reynolds in Dunsmuir, where I had so enjoyed my introduction to general practice and mountain medicine six years earlier. We were then a family of five, with three young sons: Matt at 4, Cal, 3, born in Arcadia during internship, and Sabin, born in Santa Rosa during residency, at 2. We had little money, and had to find our community for practice sooner than later.

Siskiyou County is the second largest county in California geographically, but sparsely settled, with a total population then of about 40,000. Mount Shasta had a 28-bed hospital serving the south County's 20,000 people and its three surrounding towns—Dunsmuir 8 miles south, Weed 9 miles north, and McCloud 12 miles east. There were 9 GPs collectively in those towns, all on the hospital staff.

I found out from Bill that one of the Mount Shasta physicians was in the hospital with a malignant brain tumor and would not be able to resume practice. Gene and I liked the look of the town, the area, the schools, and it was not too far from her family in Marin County, so we decided to settle there.

Knowing nothing about "practice management" (which was nowhere in graduate medical education at the time), I bought the practice from the physician's wife—for $3,500—which included good will and a 3X5 card file of patient records (often with years of "records" on each side of the card!). I rented his small office in an arcade on the main street of town.

We settled into a tract house on the outskirts of town, with a good view of Mt. Shasta from the back yard. With some help with childcare, Gene was able to resume teaching first-grade in the elementary school.

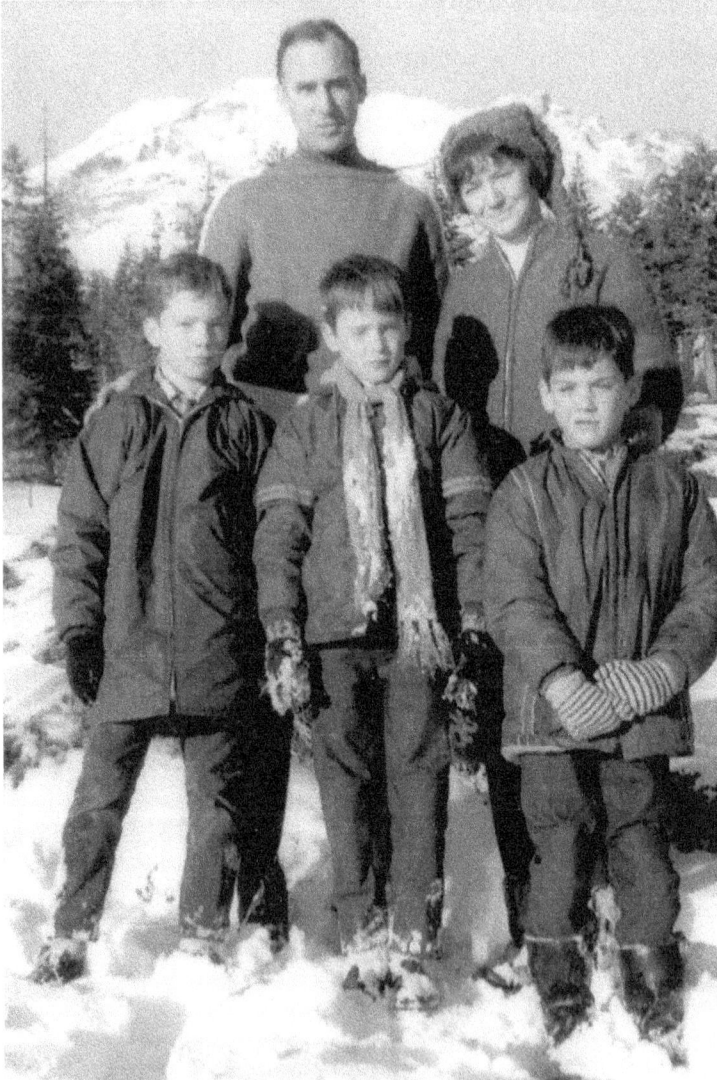

Our family in Mount Shasta, 1964

Those six years were great for the family and me. I thrived on my practice, especially being able to provide a broad range of clinical skills, being on the front lines, and continuity of care with patients and their families. No day or night was ever the same, and it was total immersion in the community, usually working 60 to 80 hours a week. All of the area's physicians were in solo practice, and the only call system was for one of us to be on call for the hospital's ER for a week at a time, Friday to Friday. The ethos was still one of rugged individualism in a rural area.

All of the other physicians had had at least two or three years of graduate training after medical school. After internships, some took a year of internal medicine and a year of surgery, while others completed a two-year general practice residency. As a result, we could learn from each other as well as from visiting consultants and the continuing medical education (CME) programs we could arrange. When we needed help, our closest referral centers were Redding, 65 miles to the south and Medford, OR, 60 miles to the north.

Each physician had his own office, usually with two or three office staff (far cry from today's staff support!). Our staffs typically included a receptionist and a nurse. We had to set up a simple accounting system and get accounting help along the way. A solo office would usually include a waiting room, reception area, two or three examination rooms, a small office laboratory, and often an x-ray machine (I would take and develop the films). Beyond those needs, we would use the hospital's facilities.

Meanwhile, we as a family enjoyed small community life which neither Gene nor I had previously had. Our boys had a good experience in the local school, we all enjoyed the country, learned to ski, and found the community supportive. After two years in the tract, we built a house three miles west of town bordering on two streams, with an acre for pasturing Gene's horse, and with a great view of Mt. Shasta.

Mount Shasta had been settled by people from northern Italy in the late 1800s, who were attracted as loggers to mountainous country they had known. We had three logging mills in town during the 1960s (all gone now), and were also on the railroad (Southern Pacific since the 1800s). The freeway, now Interstate 5, had bypassed Dunsmuir and Mount Shasta just before the 1960 World's Fair in Seattle. The area had not yet been discovered by more affluent people from the city, and life was tough for many. This was before Medicare and Medicaid, which were enacted in 1965. The reimbursement for the average office visit had just been increased from $4.00 to $5.00, while obstetrical care, including prenatal care, delivery and postpartum care, was $150.00.

Some patient vignettes will give you an idea of what practice was like in those days.

One day I got a call from a family who lived in town. Their mother might have died, "Come quick!" I left my full waiting room, charged over to their house, and found their mother supine on the floor of a wine cellar in a dark basement without lights. She was unresponsive, and the family was looking on terrified. Sitting down on the floor, I checked her vital signs—blood pressure 120/80, heart rate 80 and regular, couldn't see respirations, no obvious breath sounds, but she was fully clothed and motionless. No response to pain reflex, repeat vital signs the same, so I sat back and told the family that she will be OK. Five or ten minutes later, she started to rouse, we got her upstairs to the living room, where a further history revealed that her oldest daughter, age 18, would be leaving for college in Chico the next morning, no more than 75 miles to the south.

That was a graphic example of panic disorder and family dynamics that had not been obvious to me earlier although I had seen her on some previous occasions for headaches and other functional complaints. This was a close family, and she was going to "lose" her daughter.

Another incident got me more interested in behavioral medicine, which had not been a strong part of my earlier medical education.

> *I had seen a young woman from Doris, a very small logging community on Highway 97 between Weed and Klamath Falls, for ulcerative colitis. After several office visits, she responded well to medication. But it soon became clear that she was very depressed, as perhaps many women would be in such an isolated area, even with the use of anti-depressants such as they were at the time. I read that another GP in an Oregon town was doing marital therapy, even scheduling sessions as he would a surgical procedure. So I read the best book I could find on the subject, started trying to schedule such sessions, but never succeeded in getting both parties in the same room at the same time. This was a culture where men would not admit their role in marital problems; many were loggers and would say that they were too busy to come in.*

The Mount Shasta years were times to expand my skills and horizons. First was getting my pilot's license. After seeing a sign on the freeway south of San Francisco during medical school—"Learn to fly for $99"—I took seven hours of flight instruction, soloed, but then ran out of money. I renewed instruction in 1964, got my license, and started flying, an avocation that would turn out to be life long. Isolated as we were in Mount Shasta, I could fly to meetings in cities, take the family on visits too far to drive, and even fly down to Redding to assist on one of my patient's surgeries.

Another change that started in Mount Shasta was a new interest in how the healthcare system works—or does not work. With the advent of Regional Medical Programs (RMP—known as the Heart, Cancer, Stroke legislation of the mid-1960s), coronary care units (CCUs) were being set up all over the country and achieving remarkable outcomes of saved lives. I wanted to bring a two-bed CCU to our small rural hospital, and flew down to Sacramento for a four consecutive weekend course in coronary care. After training a dedicated group of nurses, we established such a unit and also had many remarkable saves. [1]

Other efforts did not go so well. We had no coordinated ambulance system in southern Siskiyou County. Each of the four communities had their own ambulance, not too well equipped, staffed by volunteers from their Fire Departments, who did not talk to each other. Instead, they would compete against each other as their high school football teams did. So we established a committee with representatives from each town to resolve the problem—with no positive outcomes until sometime in the early 1970s when a better organized ambulance system was finally put together.

Another step ahead for me was learning how to write. As a Geology major in college, I was a slow reader and an unskilled writer. But writing became a way to share in the larger system in a useful way. This patient vignette gave me a starting point:

> *A twenty-one-year-old woman came in for her first prenatal visit. I noticed that her eyes (the sclerae) looked a bit blue. That reminded me of osteogenesis imperfecta, which I had never seen but heard about in medical school. I called my OB/GYN consultant in Redding and a fellow*

in the OB/GYN Department at UCSF. Neither could tell me what to expect different in prenatal care, delivery, or care of the newborn. Well before the Internet, there was also no Abridged Index Medicus available to me. So I flew down to San Francisco, spent a day in the UCSF Library, researched the questions, and learned enough to proceed to a normal delivery with good outcomes for mother and baby. There was so little available in literature for clinicians that, after reading how such reports were best put together, I wrote up a case report for California Medicine. [2] *That experience launched me on a path toward future writing projects, most of which have been oriented to how local or national health care systems could work better.*

I was enjoying practice as Gene enjoyed teaching, the boys were doing fine in school, we had climbed Mt. Shasta as a family, and we had many friends in the community. Why would we think of leaving after six years? The answer came after a phone call from my good friend, Dr. Ed Neal, who, as a graduate of UCSF medical school and the Sonoma County general practice residency a year after me, was on a search committee looking for a new program director for the residency program. This would be under an RMP grant to convert the two-year general practice residency to a three-year family practice residency affiliated with UCSF. After giving it long thought, I realized that, if I stayed in practice in Mount Shasta, I would have to make changes, such as bringing in a partner. Moving back to Santa Rosa would give me a chance to participate directly in development of the new specialty, Family Practice, established in 1969, Gene could move back closer to her family, and we all had liked Santa Rosa the first time.

So that move would become our new venture, as we will see in the next chapter. But our Mount Shasta years had been formative for our family. We would go back frequently for many years thereafter to visit friends. When our sons were considering becoming engaged to their future wives, they would take them to see Mount Shasta. Gene had become a feature writer for the paper there, and taught skiing in addition to school. And I could recall many a patient's story when later passing houses in town.

Endnotes:

1. Geyman, JP. A coronary care unit in a 25-bed rural hospital. *California Medicine* 112:1, 74-77, 1970.
2. Geyman, JP. Osteogenesis imperfecta and pregnancy. *California Medicine* 107(2):171-172, 1967.

CHAPTER 16

TEACHING AND ADMINISTRATION

The Santa Rosa Years

I had always enjoyed teaching visiting medical students in the Mount Shasta practice, so this would be an exciting new venture. We made the move back to Santa Rosa in two stages—the boys, our dog, and me with a rental truck in the first stage, followed by Gene and her horse ten days later. She was able to get him in the horse trailer by herself, without much cooperation on his part, then drive 250 miles to Santa Rosa, arriving after midnight, where Dr. Scott Chilcott, a classmate from medical school and the residency, had arranged for pasturing the horse. Not wanting to cut our Mount Shasta ties completely, we rented our house to friends and kept taking the local weekly paper (for many years to come!).

Whether I wanted it or not, I was heavily involved in administration from day one back at Sonoma County Hospital. As the only full-time faculty member, I had to plan a new three-year curriculum, arrange for construction of a Family Practice Center as required for continuity practice by the residents, recruit new faculty, and set up an active affiliation with the Division of Ambulatory and Community Medicine at UCSF. The program was expanded to six residents in each of three years, strengthening broad-breadth outpatient and hospital training, including anesthesia, surgery, obstetrics-gynecology, and psychiatry. We still relied on volunteer clinical faculty from the community, but as time went on added part-time faculty in a number of specialties, periodic visiting faculty from UCSF, and an advanced surgery resident from San Francisco to help our residents with the more common, less complicated procedures.

For starters, I made a week's trip around the country to look at other new family practice residencies, both in medical schools and community programs, ranging from Kansas, Oklahoma, Florida, and South Carolina to New York. This was helpful and led to lasting friendships with colleagues. We converted our previous two-year general practice residency into a three-year family practice residency, as described in an article in *The Journal of the American Medical Association (JAMA)* in 1971. [1]

While I enjoyed teaching, especially on teaching rounds with the residents and as an attending physician in the clinic, there was little time to do it. It was difficult to realize that my direct contact with patients had gone away, especially after such a good experience in Mount Shasta. Administration was all consuming, and there was nobody else to do it. That was my job.

After two years, the program was up and running well. I realized that the biggest change toward family practice had to be in medical schools, and that leadership there had to be by real family physicians with practice experience, not academicians in other specialties without such experience. So I approached the chairman of the Division of Ambulatory and Community Medicine, a part of the Department of Medicine at UCSF, about the possibility of establishing a Department of Family Practice there. The answer was clear—no way here, too much opposition from the other specialties, and why aren't you happy with what we've already done for you?

With the brashness of a forty-year-old upstart family physician wanting to get directly involved with family practice in medical schools, I started looking around for possibilities. The University of Utah was then looking for a head of a new Division of Family

Practice within a Department of Family and Community Medicine, which had been established with solid state funding by an academic cardiologist, Dr. Hilmon Castle. Gene and I made a trip to Salt Lake City, were warmly received, liked the country, new to both of us, and decided on the move. Again, Gene always looked at the positives of a move, as she had during her childhood during the depression and war years with her own family, with 13 moves before we got married.

The University of Utah years

By 1971, about one-half of the nation's medical schools had either started or were planning family practice programs in various relationships with established clinical departments. The goal was always to achieve full departmental status, often an upward climb because of opposition from other departments, shortage of funding, and other reasons. There were about 60 family practice residency programs across the country, usually in community hospitals with or without university affiliations. The pressing need was to expand the number of these programs.

Part of the resistance to family practice in academic centers was the lack of awareness of primary care and its role in community practice. The ethos in medical schools is typically toward narrower and narrower specialization, the opposite of generalist teaching and practice. We had to develop the concepts of family medicine as an academic discipline in its own right as an area of action, with its own knowledge and clinical skills, training, and research. I tried to capture that definition in a 1971 article in *The Journal of Medical Education.* [2]

In our new Division of Family Practice, we expanded opportunities for medical students to take preceptorships with practicing family physicians in the Inter Mountain West, established a model family practice clinic at the University Medical Center, and started

217

to build a network of affiliated family practice residency programs, culminating soon with the accreditation of two such programs in Ogden at the McKay-Dee and St. Benedict's Hospitals.

Much as our family enjoyed Utah, including skiing its beautiful ski slopes, we felt a bit landlocked and were starting to miss our origins on the West coast. So we were attracted to moving back to California, where I could head up an effort to establish a large network of family practice residencies as professor and vice-chairman of a Department of Family Practice at the University of California Davis, then chaired by Dr. Len Hughes Andrus, who had had earlier primary care practice experience in the Salinas area.

The University of California Davis years

That move got Gene back closer to her family, we liked the university town of Davis, the schools were excellent, and I, as a member of the UC Davis flying club, had the whole Sacramento and San Joaquin Valleys to fly up and down to set up new affiliations for family practice residency programs.

Over the next five years, we developed a regional network of family practice residencies in four different locations—Martinez, Stockton and Merced to the south and Redding to the north. The network included new opportunities for medical student teaching as well as faculty development and continuing medical education. By the mid-1970s, there were more than 200 approved family practice residency programs across the country with 2,500 residents in these programs, two-thirds of the country's medical schools had organized departments or divisions of family practice, and student interest in the field was growing rapidly. I wrote articles describing the advantages and feasibility of starting these programs in community hospitals, [3] developing a competency-based curriculum as an organizing framework in family practice residencies [4], and the rationale, goals, components and advantages of the regional approach we were taking at UC Davis. [5]

Once again, our family was enjoying being in Davis, Gene had become a professional puppeteer, the boys were thriving in school, so why would we consider yet another move? The answer this time, was that the chairmanship of the six-year old Department of Family Medicine at the University of Washington in Seattle had come open. My friend and colleague, Dr. Ted Phillips, who had been a GP in Sitka, Alaska in the 1960s when I had been in Mount Shasta, had started the department. I was encouraged to look at the opportunity, was recruited there, and our family found our new home in Bellevue just across Lake Washington from the University.

The University of Washington years

As the only medical school over the four-state WAMI region (Washington, Alaska, Montana and Idaho), representing about one-quarter of the nation's land area, the University of Washington School of Medicine had a unique opportunity to train physicians for this region. With federal funding and the strong support of Dr. Bob Van Citters as Dean and Dr. Jack Lein as Associate Dean, the WAMI program had a dynamic start during the early 1970s. The first-year medical school class provided slots from each of the three outlying states, with the hope that graduates would later return to their home states and meet the needs for physicians, especially in more rural areas. Medical student clerkships (six-week teaching periods with practicing family physicians) were started across the WAMI area ranging from Anchorage and Juneau in Alaska to Boise, Idaho and Kalispell, Montana as well as from Seattle to Anacortes, Whidbey Island, and Spokane in Washington.

Family Medicine played a leading role as the medical school developed its new medical student, resident and continuing medical education across the WAMI region. Ted Phillips had done an excellent job in leading the Department of Family Medicine over its first six years. A clinical and teaching base was established at the University Medical Center, together with a Family Physician Pathway as one of four pathways available to students in their last two years of medical school for WAMI clerkships. In addition, a network of three-year family practice residency programs was established at four Seattle hospitals, as well as in Yakima, Spokane, and Boise, Idaho.

When I arrived at the end of 1976, the basic groundwork for the Department was well established. But, of course, there was still plenty to do. One of the next challenges was to start a Family Medicine Inpatient Service at University Hospital, whereby our faculty and residents could admit and follow their own patients in the same way that other clinical departments did. There was initially some opposition from the other departments, especially internal medicine and obstetrics-gynecology. That withered away as our faculty and residents demonstrated their competency, and as time went on, the family medicine residents were especially welcomed by the other services because of their broader clinical competencies.

Another early need was to develop the research capabilities of departmental faculty. With the support of a faculty development grant from the Robert Wood Johnson Foundation, and with Ted's leadership in a new role, this area took shape, later resulting in one of the country's major Rural Health Research Centers as well as published research in other areas related to clinical strategies, health care services, and educational methods.

Student interest in family medicine grew exponentially, at one point in the later 1980s peaking with one-third of graduating medical students at UW selecting family medicine residencies. Our network of student clerkships grew in both community-based group practices and residency programs while the residency network expanded from seven programs with 102 residents in the late 1970s to 12 programs with 185 residents in 1990. To meet the teaching needs across these networks, the number of clinical faculty across the WAMI region expanded to 130 in 1977 to more than 300 in 1990, while our full-time university-based faculty grew from 9 to more than 20.

By 1990, twenty-one years after family practice was recognized as the 20th specialty in medicine, these were some of the markers of impressive progress nationally:

- Clinical departments of family practice (not administrative departments as in earlier years) in more than one-half of departmentalized U.S. hospitals.
- Active clinical departments of family practice in most medical schools.
- More than 40,000 board-certified family physicians.
- Geriatrics as a new certifiable area of added qualifications through two certifying Boards—Internal Medicine and Family Practice.
- Family practice in high demand, with leading role in managed care.
- Academic departments of family practice in almost 90 percent of U.S. medical schools.
- 384 family practice residency programs with about 7,300 residents in training.
- Active research in many academic departments of family practice, as well as some collaborative research networks involving community settings.
- Some family medicine representation on National Institutes of Health (NIH) study sections and panels, together with 18 individuals from family medicine elected to the Institute of Medicine. [6]

I did not know in 1990 that the next 25 years would bring

remarkable further progress, especially at Sonoma County's Santa Rosa Residency and the University of Washington's Department of Family Medicine . It was gratifying to visit both places in 2015 to find that:

- The original Community Hospital of Sonoma County that opened in 1938 has evolved to a new larger hospital, Sutter Medical Center, a leading clinical and teaching center serving the larger community with an expanded residency program with 36 residents. Its graduates comprise almost one-half of the family physicians in Sonoma County, and it continues a strong affiliation with UCSF for undergraduate and graduate medical education. It continues a tradition of teaching general and family practice for more than 65 years based on the four pillars we discussed in Chapter 14. [7]

- At the University of Washington, the Department of Family Medicine has grown to a major clinical and teaching department in the medical school with 92 full-time university based faculty, more than 1,150 clinical faculty across WWAMI (which now includes Wyoming); the regional family medicine residency network has expanded to 24 programs with 539 graduates in 2015; new programs in rural practice have been started, including a Targeted Rural Underserved Track (TRUST) and the Rural Underserved Opportunities Program (RUOP); accredited fellowships are being maintained in sports medicine, integrative medicine, geriatrics, palliative care, ultrasound, academic medicine, and health policy; the Northwest Physician Assistant Program (MEDEX) has been brought into the Department; research has become a dynamic part of the Department with grant income of $3 million a year; and the Department has maintained its record over 25 years of being rated by *U.S. News and World*

Report as # 1 in the country in family medicine, while the medical school is rated # 1 in rural medicine. [8]

By 1990, after 14 years of chairing the Department, I was again looking for a new chapter. Our sons were then grown, out of college on their own, our house was oversized, and Gene and I longed to return to small community life, such as we had experienced in Mount Shasta. Before we get to that story, however, we need to talk about another area that I'd been attracted to since starting my teaching and administrative years—writing and medical publishing, which we'll turn to in the next chapter.

Endnotes:

1. Geyman, JP. Conversion of the general practice residency to family practice. *JAMA* 215:11, 1802-1807, 1971.

2. Geyman, JP. Family Medicine as an academic discipline. *Journal of Medical Education* 46: 815-820, 1971.

3. Geyman, JP. Family practice residencies in community hospitals. Supplement. *American Family Physician*, 1-9, 1974.

4. Geyman, JP. A competency-based curriculum as an organizing framework in family practice residencies. *Journal of Family Practice*, 1:1, 1974.

5. Geyman, JP. A developing regional network residency program in family practice. *Western Journal of Medicine* 121: 514-520, 1974.

6. Geyman, JP. Family medicine as an academic discipline: progress, challenges, and opportunities. *Journal of Family Practice* 31 (3): 297-303, 1990.

7. Flinders, R. *The Santa Rosa Reader: A Personal Anthology from the Family Medicine Residency (1968-2011).* Sonoma County Medical Association, 2012, pp. 76-77.

8. Norris, TE. Chair's Notes. University of Washington Department of Family Medicine. Winter 2015 Newsletter. 2015.

CHAPTER 17

WRITING, EDITING, AND
MEDICAL PUBLISHING

Writing, editing, and medical publishing were the last things I thought I would ever do when I went into medicine. As I confessed earlier, I was a slow reader in college, not skilled in writing, and didn't spend much time in libraries. But that first small case report, followed by several articles during my Mount Shasta practice years, got me started and I found that I could learn to write by reading good writing and having something to say that was worth sharing with my colleagues.

Writing in general practice at the time was limited, at least in this country. Though I never met them, two early mentors for me were Dr. Ward Darley, a leader in the American Academy of General Practice in the 1950s and advocate for its Board certification as a specialty, who had this to say:

> *It is discouraging, at least to me, that the medical profession has not yet developed a conceptual rallying point around which our system of medical care can pay more attention to one of these parts—continuing comprehensive care of patients and their ills and also of people and their health.* [1]

And across the pond in England, Dr. Patrick Byrne, professor of general practice for many years at the University of Manchester, would emphasize: "If you haven't written it down, it didn't happen."[2]

I was fortunate to be in on the ground floor of the development of a generalist field, the traditional base of health care for centuries, as a specialty in its own right. The tasks ahead were daunting—how to describe the specialty, its range of clinical competency, curricula for training programs for medical students and residents, and its areas and approaches to research in this new (but old and largely unresearched) discipline.

An early task was to define family practice as an academic discipline. It is unique among specialties in medicine as cutting across all other clinical disciplines as a generalist field encompassing the care of patients of all ages regardless of their presenting complaints. General internal medicine and general pediatrics come the closest to the generalist approach, but they are limited to age groups of patients. General practice had been integrated into medical schools elsewhere, especially in the United Kingdom, so we could draw on the work of leaders there to build our own definition of family practice as an academic discipline. Professor Ian McWhinney, widely respected clinician, teacher and philosopher in general practice, first in England and later as the first chairman of the Department of Family Medicine at the University of Western Ontario in Canada, defined family medicine by these four criteria:

1. "A distinguishable body of knowledge,
2. A unique field of action,
3. An active area of research, and
4. A training which is intellectually rigorous." [3]

He also believed that family medicine can only really be learned in a family practice, and that family practice should be taught by family physicians. [4]

Since family medicine was taking its new place in U.S. medical schools from the early 1970s on, other clinical departments were always wondering what family physicians do and how they would fit in to their already well-defined territories. All this gave me personal motivation to help define what we were up to and how we could complement otherwise neglected areas of clinical practice, teaching, and research. It was clear that this process required the written word.

In my first article for a major educational journal, written during my first year in Santa Rosa as the residency program director, I wrote that family medicine is "the only field in medicine which directs itself primarily to the total health needs of the patient and his/her family, with emphasis on the management of about 90 percent of these needs and integration of health services with the least degree of fragmentation." [5]

Writing was starting to become easier for me, and with regular practice, was also fun to help fill the void of literature in our new specialty. My next project, written by hand on our kitchen table at night and on weekends during our Santa Rosa years, was the book, *The Modern Family Doctor and Changing Medical Practice.* [6] It was not a great book, but it was the first of its kind in this country. I sent it away to some big publishers in the East, where several rejected it until David Stires, then president of Appleton Century Crofts in New York City, the second largest publisher in the U.S., surprisingly accepted it. David had grown up in a small town in Ohio where his father was a general practitioner, and knew well how important this change in medical education and practice was.

The next project was obvious—to start a peer-reviewed scientific journal in family practice. With little tradition for research, family practice in this country did not have such a journal reporting original work in the field. Our largest medical organization, the American Academy of General Practice, did have a monthly medical journal, *GP* (which in later years became *American Family Physician*), but it was largely derivative in nature, with mostly summary review articles drawing from clinical work in other specialties. The work that generalist physicians were doing in their everyday practices was not being studied and reported.

After sketching out the need for such a journal and how we might get it started, I proposed the idea to David Stires at Appleton-Century-Crofts, who again saw its potential. Drawing from some of the early leaders in family practice whom I had met during my trip across the country looking at exemplary teaching programs, we convened an organizational meeting in San Francisco in 1973.

That was our start. We established our editorial office in my office at the University of California Davis, recruited a sizable peer reviewer group and a multi-disciplinary Editorial Advisory Board, and started to seek out original work in the field. We decided initially to publish quarterly, with our first issue in May 1974. Here are some of my comments in my opening editorial:

> *There are many gaps in our existing literature. For example, we know very little about the family as a unit of care, about the natural history of common primary care problems, about the cost-effectiveness of specific health maintenance approaches, or how best to integrate the principles of behavioral science in the care of individuals and their families. The literature has generally been more disease-oriented than problem-oriented. The clinical and decision-making process of the family physician has received inadequate attention. Few articles are derived from the family physician's particular perspective. . . .*
>
> *The Journal of Family Practice is conceived as a scholarly publication that will take an honest and unbiased approach in developing an expanded literature base for this specialty. [7]*

Dr. Gayle Stephens, formerly a family physician and Residency Program Director at Wesley Medical Center in Wichita, Kansas and then Dean of the School of Primary Medical Care at the University of Alabama in Huntsville, added this comment in our opening issue:

> *I think I can speak for all family practice faculty in warmly welcoming The Journal of Family Practice as a necessary accoutrement to the academic discipline of Family Medicine. A body of literature must be developed if the discipline is to negotiate successfully the adolescent "growing pains" to become a mature and established branch of knowledge.* [8]

These are some topics in the Table of Contents of our first issue, which we called *JFP* among us, now 42 years old:

- The Future of Family Practice in Our Medical Schools
- On the Teaching and Learning of Clinical Wisdom
- Peer Review of a Small Group Practice
- A Competency-based Curriculum in Family Practice Residencies
- A Survey of Psychiatric Care in Family Practice
- An Integrated System for the Recording and Retrieval of Medical Data in a Primary Care Setting
- Primary Care Research in a Model Family Practice Unit

We started *JFP* on a subscription basis, but soon found that would not cover its start-up costs. We then shifted to controlled circulation, whereby we mailed copies to all practicing general and family physicians in the country. That of course allowed us to accept advertising, which developed quickly, but we retained full editorial control and didn't let conflicts of interest creep into our journal. Our content had to be critically peer reviewed and what we published had to meet these criteria: new, true, comprehensible, and important to our readership.

Those early years of journal editing were exciting ones. Although we invited some articles, we depended in large measure on contributions coming in over the transom reflecting original work in the new specialty in clinical, teaching and research areas. One wall of our small journal office was filled by a blackboard, where we chalked out the contents of future issues. Any day during the early years when we received several submissions was like Christmas!

Over the years of my editorship of *JFP* (1973-1990), we went through five changes of ownership from Appleton-Century-Crofts, including Lippincott, Simon and Schuster, and Meredith Corporation. Each change brought with it increased scrutiny by the accountants as to how much more money the new owner could make from this publication. We were pushed by our corporate owners to publish special issues as supplements, which the publishers gamed to their economic interests. An example of how that might have worked—the Publisher would convene a one or two day meeting of invited people to discuss drug therapy for a certain problem, pay them well, put them up in a nice place just before a major medical meeting of a family practice organization, gather their papers up and propose that *JFP* publish them. I would never publish such a supplement without inviting potential authors ourselves and full peer review. Holding to our editorial principles, we made great progress over the years as *JFP* contributed to a growing literature base in the field, though successive publishers found me more of a thorn than an asset to their business plans.

After 17 years with *JFP*, encompassing my years at UC Davis and the University of Washington, the last publisher moved on to another editor, while I was asked to become the second editor of the *Journal of the American Board of Family Practice* (now the *Journal of the American Board of Family Medicine),* which had been started as a peer reviewed journal by the Board some years previously. I did that for another 13 years, making 30 years in total of journal editing. I enjoyed that entire experience, and it is gratifying that both journals are alive and well today, together with two other journals in the field, *Family Medicine* and the *Annals of Family Medicine*.

Writing, editing, and later publishing, all went together for me, each supporting the skills needed for the others. Editing made me a rapid reader for content, broadened my awareness of what was happening in our specialty, and further improved my writing by seeing better writing by others. Journal editing made me more aware of the changing economic pressures on publishers and the revolution taking place—including growth of Amazon, decline of bookstores, consolidation among publishers, changing readership patterns, arrival of Kindles and e-books, and growth of social media. Most journals became ever more dependent on advertising, which in turn could lead to pressure on editors to restrict the publication of some articles that were seen as threatening the economic hold of corporate publishers on their financial bottom lines.

In 1990, I turned full-time to research and writing on the health care system. With Gene's support and encouragement, each new focus resulted in a book, ranging from the corporate transformation of health care, the safety net, the privatization of Medicare, the corrosion of medicine and its moral legacy, the workings of the private health insurance industry, and the primary care crisis. In 2012, I turned to the politics and aftermath of the Affordable Care Act. As with journal writing, I found over recent years that most large publishers, owned as they are by corporate interests, shy away from books that might threaten the business model of publishing and the status quo of a profit-driven health care system. As an example, I jumped through all of the hoops required by *Publisher's Weekly* in advance of publication of my 2015 book, *How Obamacare Is Unsustainable: Why We Need a Single-Payer Solution for All Americans,* but their staff still ended up "declining to consider it."

Because of these kinds of experiences, I formed my own small, independent publishing firm, Copernicus Healthcare with a different kind of mission. As we recall, Nicolaus Copernicus (1473-1543) was a Renaissance astronomer who conceived a comprehensive heliocentric cosmology that, for the first time, displaced the Earth from the center of the universe, instead putting the sun in that center. This became a landmark and paradigm shift in the history of science. Copernicus Healthcare sees a Copernican shift now needed in U.S. health care, as shown in Figure 17.1, which can turn around our thinking in health care by 180 degrees in these ways:

- "Move stakeholders in the medical-industrial complex from the center of our 'system', and replace them with patients and their families.
- Explore how today's fragmented and depersonalized health care can be shifted towards more personal caring and healing relationships between caregivers and patients.
- Move from profits driven by a business 'ethic' to a not-for-profit system based on service.
- Shift from a system based on ability to pay to one based on medical need.
- Move from health care as a commodity for sale on a free market to a basic human need and right.
- Move from a dysfunctional, fragmented and exploitive private health insurance industry to a single publicly-financed risk pool.
- Move from political and lobbyist-driven coverage policies toward those based on scientific evidence of cost-effectiveness.
- Replace today's unaccountable system with one that stewards limited health care resources for the benefit of all Americans ('Everybody in, nobody out.')." [9]

FIGURE 17.1

COPERNICAN PARADIGM SHIFT
IN HEALTH CARE

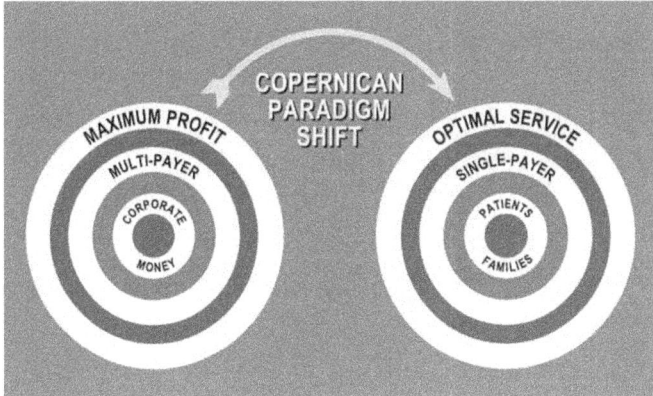

Since the start of Copernicus Healthcare, we have been glad to publish books leading to better health care and social justice, including Dr. Quentin Young's book, *Everybody In Nobody Out: Memoirs of a Rebel Without a Pause*, and Dr. Joshua Freeman's *Health, Medicine and Justice: Designing a Fair and Equitable Healthcare System*.

Surprising as it might seem from where I started in the 1960s in family medicine, writing has become a passion for me, which raises the question of why we write. It is, after all, considerable work and very time-consuming. In a 2013 article for the journal *Family Medicine*, I answered that question for me this way:

1. *To learn more than we know at the start of a writing project and to share new knowledge with our readers.*
2. *To advance our specialty and to add new information that is true, important, and of value to our readers.*
3. *To examine questions or issues related to our profession and the health of the public.*
4. *To clarify complicated subjects by cutting through to the essentials.*

5. *To bear witness to the problems being faced by our patients during the current health care crisis.*

6. *To expose conflicts of interest that run counter to our patients' interests, and*

7. *To advance the public good.*

Or to sum all that up: "We write to shine a bright light on a better future for our patients and our profession." [10]

Endnotes:

1. Darley, W. Medical education and comprehensive medical care. *GP 32*: 166, 1965.

2. Byrne, P. As quoted by Geyman, JP. Why do we write? *Family Medicine* 45 (1): 40, 2013.

3. McWhinney, IR. General practice as an academic discipline. *Lancet*, February, 419-423, 1966.

4. Frey, JJ, Ventres, WB. Voices from family medicine: Ian McWhinney. *Family Medicine* 24; 317-320, 1992.

5. Geyman, JP. Family medicine as an academic discipline. *Journal of Medical Education* 46: 815-820, 1971.

6. Geyman, JP. *The Modern Family Doctor and Changing Medical Practice*. New York. *Appleton-Century-Crofts*, 1971.

7. Geyman, JP. Expanded literature base as a critical need in family practice. *J. Fam Pract* 1:1: 4, 1974.

8. Stephens, G. Toward a body of literature in family medicine. *J Fam Pract* 1: 1: 5, 1974. Copernicus Healthcare.

9. Putting care and justice into healthcare. www.copernicus.healthcare.org

10. Geyman, JP. Why do we write? *Family Medicine* 45 (1): 40-41, 2013.

CHAPTER 18

RETURN TO RURAL PRACTICE

In 1990, after 20 years in cities during our university teaching years, Gene and I were missing small community life. After 14 years chairing the Department of Family Medicine at the University of Washington, it was time to turn the reins over to another leader for its next stage of development. So we started looking around for a small community with needs for a family physician within an hour or so from Seattle. And of course, that community had to have an airport!

When we found the San Juan Islands, specifically Friday Harbor on San Juan Island, we knew this would be the place. It was a town of about 2,500, the same size as Mount Shasta, had a clinic needing another family physician, had a good airport with an instrument approach, and was the County seat for some 17,000 people spread across a number of islands with a tradition of service-oriented health care.

We soon found our house on the west side of San Juan Island. We could see south across the water to the Olympic Mountains and eight miles west to Victoria, BC on Vancouver Island just across the U.S.-Canadian border, as well as Mt. Rainier some 140 miles southeast on a clear day. As all of our previous decisions about where to land, this decision was almost immediate and completely shared.

While I was glad to get back to practicing family medicine and being part of the community, Gene once again became active in community activities, including some substitute teaching, puppeteering, working as an EMT, and helping out with the County Fair.

Rural Health Care in the San Juan Islands

Like most somewhat isolated rural communities, the San Juan Islands had trouble recruiting and retaining physicians. They had benefitted greatly from the long career of Dr. Malcolm Heath, who had, from his base in Friday Harbor, served the islands as a generalist physician for some 30 years after World War II, including also as the county health officer. There was no call system, and he was available night and day. He learned to fly, and flew regularly to Bellingham, WA, 25 miles away on the mainland, to deliver his obstetric patients.

In 1955, the Inter-Island Medical Center (IIMC) was established on San Juan Island by interested members of the community. While patients were welcomed from neighboring islands, transportation was limited by ferry schedules. As a result, in later years, some physicians came to practice on the nearby Orcas and Lopez islands.

The IIMC in Friday Harbor was governed and owned by a community board of directors, renting office space to Dr. Heath but making no attempt to manage his practice. With the advent of a Hill-Burton loan from the federal government in 1976, a new facility was built to hospital specifications, with payback of the loan by providing free care to the poor for a period of 20 years. As Hill-Burton also required, the IIMC purchased the assets of Dr. Heath's medical practice, and physicians from then on would be employees of the IIMC as the board undertook all aspects of its management.

As would be expected, it took three physicians to fill Dr. Heath's shoes when he retired in 1978. The island's population was growing and later physicians expected coverage in rotation for after-hours care. The 1980s saw a revolving door of physicians, recurrent financial shortfalls of the IIMC, strife over its governance between the board, which attempted to micromanage the practice, and the physicians, resulting in some volatility of board membership. Reimbursement for patient care services from payers was low, as is typical in rural practice, especially since this was a clinic without licensed inpatient beds or an emergency room, and not being operated as a hospital. Extensive and life-saving services were often provided for hours, or even overnight, for acutely ill patients with such problems as heart attacks and diabetic ketoacidosis, especially when weather precluded emergency transport to a mainland hospital. Such care could never be compensated at the level of routine office visits.

The crisis came to a head in 1989, when a deficit of $324,500 forced an announcement that the IIMC's doors would have to be closed unless a solution could be found. The IIMC had been losing about $100,000 a year in contractual losses, including Medicare, Medicaid, and Hill-Burton sources. After a heated and controversial debate, progressive leadership within the community fortunately led to the formation of a tax-supported hospital district board such as had occurred in several other rural communities for these kinds of reasons. There was strong community support for continuation of the wide range of medical services that they had enjoyed for years, and the hospital district was passed by an 80 percent vote. A local property tax was levied that amounted to about $150 of additional tax for families owning property of $200,000 assessed valuation. That tax support saved the IIMC for a number of years, although its financial woes were to re-appear in later years. The genesis of the hospital district was described in a 1994 article, including lessons to be learned from the problems it helped to resolve at the time. [1] During most of my practice years in the 1990s, our three-FTE family practice was relatively stable, especially with the leadership of Dr. David Gimlett, who combined clinical expertise with management skills, including evolving the practice to computers. We served our island and some of the smaller islands with a regular call schedule

24-hours a day, 7 days-per-week. As family physicians, we had a broad breadth of clinical skills, including emergency care, internal medicine, pediatrics, orthopedics, and geriatrics. We all had training in obstetrics-gynecology, but did not do deliveries on the island, since we were not prepared for possible Caesarian sections and lacked blood if the need for transfusions arose. Instead, we shared prenatal care with physicians on the mainland who would do the deliveries. The IIMC was fully equipped as an emergency care facility, with necessary laboratory, radiographic, and support services typical of the times.

We had a close working relationship with Emergency Medical Services, which was well organized under the leadership of Frank Wilson, EMT and veteran of the Vietnam War. As one example of our excellent EMS service, we did a study of out-of-hospital cardiac arrests on the island from 1978 to 1994, finding that our survival rates, including neurological outcomes six months later, were comparable to those in Seattle, where Medic One was started, and better than any other reports from rural areas. The reasons for our good outcomes were largely because of quick response times by EMTs and paramedics, who had defibrillators available from the start. [2] Other medical services on the island included an 85-bed convalescent center next to the IIMC, a mental health counseling center, one general internist in solo practice, and regularly visiting specialists to the IIMC from the mainland.

During these practice years, I was also still active at the University, flying there once or twice a week to keep involved with my editorial work with the Board journal and staying in touch with some other activities in the Department of Family Medicine. That was not really work, since I got to fly both ways, often landing on floats on Portage Bay right next to the campus and walking to work!

Two things happened in 1997 that led me to decide to stop clinical practice, at age 66, much as I was enjoying it. I wanted to spend more time doing research and writing on the health care system. Staying involved with patient care prevented that. By 1997, it was also time to turn the editorship of the *Journal of the American Board of Family Medicine* over to Dr. Marjorie Bowman at Wright State University in Dayton, Ohio. Both decisions lead us to the next chapter.

Endnotes:

1. Taplin, SE, Geyman, JP, Gimlett, D. Family practice and the health care system. The public hospital district for ambulatory care: an option to stabilize rural health services in crisis. *Journal of the American Board of Family Practice.* 7: 493-502, 1994.

2. Killien, SY, Geyman, JP, Gossom, JB, Gimlett, D. Out-of-hospital cardiac arrest in a rural area: A sixteen year experience with lessons learned and national comparisons. *Annals of Emergency Medicine* 28 (3): 294-300, 1996.

CHAPTER 19

THE POST-PRACTICE YEARS:

Changing Political Perspectives and Advocacy for Reform

It is perfectly true, as philosophers say, that life must be understood backward, but they forget the other proposition, that it must be lived forward.

—Soren Kierkegaard

With new block time available after leaving clinical practice, my vista was wide open to examine and write about what seemed to me to be a failing health care system increasingly more concerned about profits than care of patients. I now had time to read more widely and explore what was happening in different parts of the system.

In 1980, Dr. Arnold Relman, internist and former editor of *The New England Journal of Medicine*, noted the emergence of a medical-industrial complex, an expanding new for-profit industry ranging from proprietary hospitals and nursing homes to diagnostic services, medical devices, hemodialysis, the pharmaceutical industry, the insurance industry, home care, and many other related proprietary activities. He gave us this warning 36 years ago:

This new "medical-industrial complex" may be more efficient than its not-for-profit competition, but it creates the problems of overuse and fragmentation of services, overemphasis on technology, and "cream skimming," and it may also exercise undue influence on national health policy. Closer attention from the public and the profession, and careful study are necessary to ensure that the "medical-industrial complex" puts the interests of the public before those of its stockholders. [1]

At the close of the 1990s, this warning seemed to me all too evident. In the managed care era of the 1990s, mostly for-profit HMOs were being discredited as restricting access to necessary care as they sought greater profits from supposedly managing care for a defined population. The more patients they could contract for on an annual basis, in their terms "covered lives," the higher their financial returns. The growth of investor-owned, for-profit chains, started in the 1960s, was gaining momentum in a largely unregulated market, while the health insurance industry was following the trends among hospitals and HMOs—mergers, consolidation, and oligopoly. Insurers were emphasizing medical underwriting, considered unethical before the 1970s, in their efforts to avoid higher-risk patients— avoiding the sick and covering the healthy for greater revenues. Meanwhile, prices and costs were increasing in related industries, such as pharmaceuticals, medical devices, nursing homes, mental health facilities, and dialysis centers, that were making health care more unaffordable for a growing part of the population. [2] By 2002, there were 41 million Americans without health insurance. [3]

My first book to look at the whole health care system, in 2002, was *Health Care in America: Can Our Ailing System Be Healed?* As I wrote in its preface:

That widespread turmoil exists in the organization, financing, and delivery of health care in the United States as we enter the 21ˢᵗ Century is beyond doubt. Health care issues have received increasing media coverage and tak-

en center stage in the politics of our time. Health care in America now represents one seventh of the world's largest economy, up from one twenty-fifth just 40 years ago. There is growing awareness, however, that size does not connote strength. Many are increasingly frustrated and unhappy with U.S. health care, whether they are patients, providers, payers, or legislators. The present system is unsustainable in the long run because of its three main problems: escalating costs, limitations of access, and wide variations in quality. An intense national debate is taking place as to how to reform or revise our health care system in public interest in a fair and sustainable way. [4]

That statement applies today 15 years later even more than then. It summarizes my growing discontent with the directions of our health care system. They are foreign to my experience in practice, both in the 1960s and 1990s, when access to affordable care was generally available and when health care and the medical profession were more service-oriented. My political views have become more progressive with a committment to better inform myself and others about possible directions to reform the system.

Before long, I became aware of the excellent work being done by Physicians for a National Health Program (PNHP), an advocacy organization of U.S. physicians, medical students and health professionals co-founded in 1986 by Drs. David Himmelstein and Steffie Woolhandler. Its mission is to educate Americans about single-payer national health insurance as a necessary approach to health care reform. Its membership has grown steadily as it established state chapters across the country. I was fortunate to meet many colleagues dedicated to real health care reform for the common good, and was privileged to serve as PNHP's president from 2005 to 2007.

Some Further Writings

My next book, in 2004, *The Corporate Transformation of Health Care: Can the Public Interest Still Be Served?*, discussed the corporatization of U.S. health care across many industries, including HMOs, hospitals, nursing homes, health insurance, the pharmaceutical industries, and other medically related industries. Ways in which health care corporations defend and promote their interests were discussed, as well as the growing threat to the public interest of investor-owned care. Here's how Drs. Woolhandler and Himmelstein, internists and co-founders of PNHP, saw the problems with investor-owned care:

> *Our main objection to investor-owned care is not that it wastes taxpayers money, not even that it causes modest decrements in quality. The most serious problem with such care is that it embodies a new value system that severs the communal roots and samaritan traditions of hospitals, makes doctors and nurses the instruments of investors, and views patients as commodities. In non-profit settings, avarice vies with beneficence for the soul of medicine; investor ownership represents the triumph of greed.* [5]

My 2005 book, *Falling Through the Safety Net: Americans Without Health Insurance*, explored the question as to how much safety net existed with 45 million uninsured Americans, and when more than one-third of people losing their jobs lost their health insurance and could not afford other coverage. More than 30 family stories and patient vignettes were described illustrating system problems that were decimating a safety net. The myth held by many conservatives that "everyone gets care anyhow" (such as through emergency rooms) was rebutted, as were other myths, such as "a general right to health care would bring a government takeover and socialized medicine" and "the free market in health care is the most fair and efficient". [6]

My interest then shifted to Medicare, which since 1965 had been a dependable program for seniors aged 65 and older. After summarizing the history of Medicare since 1965 and trends toward privatization, my 2006 book, *Shredding the Social Contract: The Privatization of Medicare,* compared claims of the privatizers with the reality of their changes. Here are two typical quotes from the book, still relevant today, that reveal the wide gulf in thinking about health insurance in this country—the first supports the idea that the government has a responsibility to provide some form of social insurance, while the second argues against any such role of government and puts individuals and families on their own:

> *One of the most striking features of Medicare's political evolution is how the ideological cleavage that attended its birth reappeared, in a different guise, more than three decades later. Most reform advocates, for obvious reasons, claim an interest in "saving Medicare." But the equally obvious truth is that the program still excites fundamental differences about the proper role of government in health insurance.*
>
> *For those who embrace its social insurance purposes, this would be satisfaction. For those who reject those principles as inappropriate, the fight over "reforming" Medicare is in fact about changing it fundamentally.*
>
> —Theodore Marmor, professor of political science and public health at Yale University and author of *The Politics of Medicare* [7]

The new (health care) system also must be responsive primarily to individual consumers rather than third-party payers, such as the government, insurers, and employers. A consumer-driven system will empower all people—if they choose—to make decisions that will directly affect the most fundamental and intimate aspect of their life—their own health. This empowerment gives people a greater stake in and more responsibility for their own health care. Health care will not improve in a sustained and substantial way until consumers drive it.

—2004 Senate Majority Leader Bill Frist,
former general and thoracic surgeon [8]

I next became aware of a growing body of literature over the preceding ten years calling attention to a wide range of conflicts of interest between many physicians and industry, a decline of public trust in the medical profession, a decrease in physicians' clinical autonomy, and demoralization within the profession. [9-13] That led me to ask what are the goals of the medical profession and whose interests should the health care system serve? That led to my 2008 book, *The Corrosion of Medicine: Can the Profession Reclaim Its Moral Legacy?*, which explores the long history of the medical profession's proud tradition of service and asks to what extent the changing profession can lead toward health care reform. I found these two contrasting views of the goals of our health care system striking, but showing how far apart ideological viewpoints are on our political spectrum: [14]

Do we have an obligation to provide health care for everybody? Where do we draw the line? Is any fast-food restaurant obligated to feed everybody who shows up?

—Richard Scott, co-founder, chairman, CEO and president, Columbia/HCA Healthcare Corporation, the largest investor-owned hospital chain in the country (who was later fired from his post when the chain was found guilty of fraud and settled for $1.7 billion), [15] and now is Governor of Florida.

Making fat profits on hospitals at the expense of the poor and the sick may not be a prison offense in this country. What is a crime is the galloping privatization of the nation's health resources and the rise of a competitive health care system that has less and less to do with health and access to care and everything to do with money.

—California Representative Pete Stark, member of the House Ways and Means health subcommittee

The more I read, studied the system, and learned, the more obvious it became to look closely at the private health insurance industry itself. My 2008 book, *Do Not Resuscitate: Why the Health Insurance Industry Is Dying, and How We Must Replace It,* was the logical sequel. Despite the claims of health insurers, this book documented these problems which made the industry unsustainable: continued escalation of uncontrolled costs of health care, continued decline of employer-sponsored insurance, less insurance coverage for higher costs, more insecurity over access to health care, more corporate lobbying and disinformation as the industry was fighting a last-ditch battle for survival. Robert Kuttner, economist, co-editor of *The American Prospect*, and author of *Everything for Sale: The Virtues and Limits of Markets*, made this prescient observation in 2006, which has now become common knowledge:

> *At no time since the Great Depression have the work-*
> *ing poor and the working middle class had more in com-*
> *mon in their economic vulnerability, or been more in need*
> *of cross-class government programs, such as reliable pen-*
> *sions, health insurance, protections against income loss,*
> *and new needs of the broadly defined working family, such*
> *as child care. To the extent that a class war is going on, it*
> *is the top 1 percent versus the bottom 80 percent.* [16]

The next big development, of course, was the battle over health care reform in 2008-2009 that finally led to passage in 2010 of the Patient Protection and Affordable Care Act (PPACA), now known simply as Obamacare or the Affordable Care Act (ACA). It has become obvious in recent years that it is misnamed, since health care in this country continues to be more expensive and less affordable, despite its benefits and subsidies. The outcome was obvious from the beginning, as described in my 2010 book, *Hijacked: The Road to Single-Payer in the Aftermath of Stolen Health Care Reform*, which describes the many ways in which corporate interests and their lobbyists wrote the legislation in their own favor. I found Bill Moyers' observation compelling about what happened:

> *This is a perilous moment. The individualist, greed-*
> *driven free market ideology that both of our major parties*
> *have pursued is at odds with what most Americans really*
> *care about. Popular support for either party has struck bot-*
> *tom, as more and more agree that growing inequality is bad*
> *for the country, that corporations have too much power, that*
> *money in politics has corrupted our system, and that work-*
> *ing families and poor communities need and deserve help*
> *because the free market has failed to generate shared pros-*
> *perity—its famous unseen hand has become a closed fist.* [17]

As a family physician, I was concerned about the decline of primary care as the nation's physician workforce was becoming more and more specialized despite impressive advances of family medicine as its own specialty. I next wanted to examine the history and trends in the decline of primary care, including how primary care could be rebuilt as the base of our system. My 2011 book, *Breaking Point: How the Primary Care Crisis Endangers the Lives of Americans*, did just that. These two takeaway points by other observers were discussed earlier in Chapter 5.

> *The 2009-10 health reform effort has addressed two interrelated crises: declining health insurance coverage, and high and rising costs. A third crisis also has captured the attention of policy makers: the decline of primary care. If the primary care foundation of the health care system is not strengthened, true access and cost containment may be impossible.* [18]

> *The U.S. government ceded [the generalist-specialist mix issue] to academic medicine and hospitals, whose leadership naturally focused on specialty-oriented research, training, and clinical care.* [19]

As more and more attention was being paid to the high costs of cancer care which an aging 79 million-strong Baby Boomer generation was facing, my next focus was to look at the impacts of system trends on patients with cancer. Over a lifetime, the American Cancer Society was telling us that 45 percent of men and 38 percent of women are expected to develop cancer. As a cancer survivor myself (metastatic testicular cancer at age 51), my interest was more than academic. My 2012 book, *The Cancer Generation: Baby Boomers Facing a Perfect Storm,* found, as expected, that the uninsured and underinsured frequently cannot afford care, and have less cancer screening, delayed diagnosis, higher mortality, and high levels of medical bankruptcy. Increasingly, oncologists were concerned about the spiraling costs of cancer care, decreasing access to care, the unsustainability of these trends, and how their practices are beset with conflicts of interest in their roles as treating physicians. Arthur Caplan, bioethics professor at the University of Pennsylvania, called this "one of the toughest issues in oncology, since drug prices can involve 'exchanging family assets' for the possibility of a few more months of life." [20]

It was becoming clear to me, as for many others, that deregulated markets were failing the object of health care—the patient. So my next book, in 2012, *Health Care Wars: How Market Ideology and Corporate Power Are Killing Americans*, examined how this was happening, with no change on the horizon. Fifty thousand Americans were dying each year for lack of health insurance, 2 million cancer patients were forgoing care due to unaffordable costs, and another 2 million were going bankrupt, despite most being insured. The case was made in this book that we are in an undeclared class war in this country over the soul and humanity of America, over the future of the middle class, and over what kind of country we are.

By 2015, with the Affordable Care Act the law of the land for five years, it was time to analyze its experience. My next book, *How Obamacare Is Unsustainable: Why We Need a Single-Payer Solution for All Americans*, attempted to cut through rhetoric, disinformation, and myths to assess its benefits and failures. In the highly polarized political environment after the 2014 midterm elections, the case for single-payer national health insurance was made in three ways—on economic, social/political, and moral grounds.

My latest book, in 2016, *The Human Face of ObamaCare: Promises vs. Reality and What Comes Next*, brings us up to date after six years' experience with the ACA. It includes more than 50 patient sto-ries that illustrate the many ways that the ACA falls short for so many millions of Americans. It compared the three main choices for health care reform during the 2016 election season—improving the ACA as needed, repealing and replacing it with a Republican plan, and a single-payer Medicare for All program of national health insurance.

Activism at the Local Level

My interest in improving health care for patients has been long-standing, including at the local level, such as trying to improve cardiac care and ambulance service in our rural county during the Mount Shasta years. So it was only natural that, when asked to join the San Juan County Board of Health, I was willing to get involved.

A major issue was starting to divide the San Juan Island com-munity. The Hospital District Board that we discussed in the last chapter, which had saved the Inter Island Medical Center (IIMC) from closing its doors in 1989, had signed a 50-year contract (with-out a public vote) with Peace Health. It is a Catholic network of hospitals ranging from Oregon to Southeast Alaska, with the closest one just 25 miles northeast across the water in Bellingham, WA.

Since the 1990s, the IIMC had continued to serve the com-munity well, but was faced with recurrent financial problems in an aging Hill-Burton facility, constrained as an ambulatory facility in billing payers for the full extent of services provided. Along came a group to remedy that problem by establishing a rural critical access hospital with newly available federal funding, together with philan-thropic contributions of some $10 million.

Peace Island Medical Center was given full charge of its op-erations, including hiring and firing of its personnel. The San Juan Hospital District Board continued to be responsible for Emergency Medical Services, but essentially handed over its oversight responsibility to Peace Health. The new 10-bed hospital had brought the island a beautiful $40-million facility, with expanded clinic space, a licensed emergency room, the latest technology for imaging procedures, and other physical improvements. But it wasn't long before it became clear that it also brought new problems—urgent care hours were restricted, the ER was being overused as a revenue center, imaging procedures were being overused, increased costs (including new facility fees) were making access unaffordable for many patients, and some reproductive services as well as Death with Dignity options were restricted under the Ethical and Religious Directives (ERDs) of the Catholic bishops.

Our elected Board of Health listened to a growing chorus of complaints from the community, attempted to understand the extent of these problems, and brought them up with the leadership of the Hospital District and PIMC. Such dialogue was not welcome, so we drew up a Patients' Bill of Rights for residents of San Juan County, which attempted to remedy some of these problems, such as gaining increased access to urgent care, making costs more affordable, making necessary and legal services available to patients without religious restrictions, and identifying the medical needs of the community with additional input from local citizens. As the community became more involved in these issues, three new members were elected to the five-person Hospital District Board, all committed to redress these problems. So real progress is in process, as it is in other Washington counties and in some other states across the country in reaction to restrictions in Catholic hospitals.

The situation with our new hospital on San Juan Island turns out, as expected, to be a microcosm of trends across the country—such as increased prices and costs of consolidating hospital systems, the business "ethic" trumping the service ethic, and backlash to restricted services in Catholic hospitals. In Washington State,

Catholic institutions account for more than 45 percent of acute-care hospital beds in the state, and bishops are vigorously enforcing the ERDs, holding their employed physicians to their adherence or loss of employment. [21,22] As discussed in Chapter 10, abortion would be expected to be restricted in Catholic facilities, but questions arise when one considers other common patients' needs, including contraception, how miscarriages or tubal pregnancies would be managed, and whether patient and family requests for legal Death with Dignity be honored. [23]

After 60 years in medicine and as a retired family physician, I continue to believe that each of us can make a difference in improving the lives of people around us—and further that physicians have a special obligation to speak out in the public interest when our health care system works against the common good, as it certainly does these days.

Now it is time to look at today's realities in our health care system, see what we can learn from its transformation, and consider directions for health care reform, as we will do in Part Three.

Endnotes:

1. Relman, AS. The new medical-industrial complex. *N Engl J Med 303*: 963-970, 1980.

2. Geyman, JP. The corporate transformation of medicine and its impact on costs and access to care. *JABFP* 16 (5): 443-454, 2002.

3. Findley, S. Bridge temporary insurance gaps. *USA Today*, September 26, Sect A: 11, 2002.

4. Geyman, JP. *Health Care in America: Can Our Ailing System Be Healed?* Boston, MA. *Butterworth Heinemann*, ix, 2002.

5. Woolhandler, S, Himmelstein, DU. Healthcare crisis and opportunity. *PNHP Newsletter,* January, 6-8, 2002:

6. Geyman, JP. *Falling Through the Safety Net: Americans Without Health Insurance.* Monroe, ME. *Common Courage Press*, 2005.

7. Marmor, TR. *The Politics of Medicare.* New York. *Aldine De Gruyter*, 2000, p. 191.

8. Frist, WH. Health care in the 21st century. *N Engl J Med* 352 (3): 267-272, 2004.

9. Rodwin, MA. *Medicine, Money & Morals: Physicians' Conflicts of Interest.* New York. *Oxford University Press*, 1993.

10. Annas, GJ. *Some Choice: Law, Medicine, and the Market.* New York. *Oxford University Press*, 1998.

11. Angell, M. *The Truth About Drug Companies: How They Deceive Us and What We Can Do About It.* New York. *Random House*, 2004.

12. Abramson, J. *Overdo$ed America: The Broken Promise of American Medicine.* New York. *Harper Collins*, 2004.

13. Kassirer, JP. *On the Take: How America's Complicity With Big Business Can Endanger Your Health.* New York. *Oxford University Press*, 2005.

14. Ginsberg, P. The patient as profit center: Hospital, Inc. comes to town. *The Nation*, November 18, 1996: 18, 22.

15. Hightower, J. Taking us for a ride on health care 'reform'. *The Progressive Populist* 15 (16), September 15, 2009, p. 3.

16. Kuttner, R. Thinking about the government. *The American Prospect* 17 (10): 3, 2006.

17. Moyers, B, Winship, M. Dr. King's economic dream deferred. *Truthout*, April 3, 2010.

18. Bodenheimer, T, Pham, HH. Primary care: current problems and proposed solutions. *Health Affairs* 29 (5): 799, 2010.

19. Sandy, LG, Bodenheimer, T, Pawlson, LG, Starfield, B. The political economy of U.S. primary care. *Health Affairs* 28 (4): 1139, 2009.

20. Chase, M. Pricey drugs put squeeze on doctors. *Wall Street Journal*, July 8, 2008: A:1.

21. Geyman, JP. Catholic hospital systems: a growing threat to access to reproductive services. *Huffington Post*, March 11, 2014.

22. Stulberg, DB, Dude, AM, Dahlquist, BS, Curlin, FA. Obstetrician-gynecologists, religious institutions, and conflicts regarding patient care policies. *Am J Obstet Gyn* 207 (1): 73, 2012.

23. Stewart, K. At Catholic hospitals, a 'right to life' but not a right to death. *The Nation*, October 8, 2015.

PART THREE

TODAY'S REALITIES AND THE FUTURE
OF U.S. HEALTH CARE

The care of human life and happiness, and not their destruction, is the first and only legitimate object of good government.

—Thomas Jefferson, in an address to the Republican
Citizens of Washington County, Maryland, March 31, 1809

The test of our progress is not whether we add more to the abundance of those who have so much; it is whether we provide enough for those who have too little.

—Franklin Delano Roosevelt
Second Inaugural Address, January 20, 1937

The only thing new in the world is the history you do not know.

—Harry S. Truman

CHAPTER 20

TODAY'S HEALTH CARE:
SO FAR SHORT OF THE NEEDS

Shouldn't we be able to expect that, as Americans, we all can get needed health care whenever we have an accident or get sick? That, in urgent or emergency situations, we can get care whatever our income or circumstances? That we won't die for lack of insurance or care? That a major illness will not bankrupt us? That health professionals, hospitals and other facilities will have our best interests at heart? That professionalism will trump self-interest? And that our health care will be at least as good as other advanced countries around the world?

These don't seem to be unreasonable expectations in a country like ours that spends about twice as much on health care as most other advanced countries. Yet these expectations are just unfulfilled dreams in the United States, in contrast to being the norm in most other advanced nations.

It is also a myth, fanned by conservatives and market advocates, that we have the best health care system in the world. This kind of view reflects an uninformed attitude of American exceptionalism. Such a claim has been discredited by many cross-national studies over many years, as illustrated by Figure 20.1, a 2014 ranking of health care systems in eleven advanced countries by the Commonwealth Fund. [1] All, except for the U.S., consider health care a human right, provide universal access to affordable health care, have better outcomes of care than we do for their whole populations, and are in sustainable, more accountable systems than we have.

FIGURE 20.1

Overall Ranking of Eleven Health Care Systems

COUNTRY RANKINGS
Top 2*
Middle
Bottom 2*

	AUS	CAN	FRA	GER	NETH	NZ	NOR	SWE	SWIZ	UK	US
OVERALL RANKING (2013)	4	10	9	5	5	7	7	3	2	1	11
Quality Care	2	9	8	7	5	4	11	10	3	1	5
Effective Care	4	7	9	6	5	2	11	10	8	1	3
Safe Care	3	10	2	6	7	9	11	5	4	1	7
Coordinated Care	4	8	9	10	5	2	7	11	3	1	6
Patient-Centered Care	5	8	10	7	3	6	11	9	2	1	4
Access	8	9	11	2	4	7	6	4	2	1	9
Cost-Related Problem	9	5	10	4	8	6	3	1	7	1	11
Timeliness of Care	6	11	10	4	2	7	8	9	1	3	5
Efficiency	4	10	8	9	7	3	4	2	6	1	11
Equity	5	9	7	4	8	10	6	1	2	2	11
Healthy Lives	4	8	1	7	5	9	6	2	3	10	11
Health Expenditures/Capita, 2011*	$3,800	$4,522	$4,118	$4,495	$5,099	$3,182	$5,669	$3,925	$5,643	$3,405	$8,508

Notes: *Includes ties, **Expenditures shown in $US PPP (Purchasing Power Parity). Australian $ data from 2010.

Source: Reprinted with permission from Davis, K, Stremikis, K, Squires, D et al. *Mirror, Mirror on the Wall, 2014 Update: How the U.S. Health Care System Compares Internationally.* The Commonwealth Fund, June 16, 2014.

As we have seen in earlier chapters, many tens of millions of Americans are left out of our existing system while denial of our crisis in health care continues without significant reform. Let's summarize where the U.S. actually is today in terms of 12 dimensions of our health care system seven years after passage of the Affordable Care Act (ACA) in 2010.

Today's Health Care Realities
1. Restricted access and choice

Access to care depends largely on an individual's insurance status and ability to pay, not medical need. The first question asked of a patient seeking care is what insurance he or she has. While the EMTALA law does require that a patient being seen in a hospital emergency room be stabilized before release, that does not assure the availability or adequacy of required follow-up care. The ACA has helped access in states that expanded Medicaid, but not in the 19 states that haven't done so. Sign-ups for ACA coverage have fallen far short of initial projections—just 11.1 million people as of March 2016 compared to an initial forecast of 24 million people. [2]

Those with insurance are finding their choices of hospital and physician severely limited by narrowed networks that can change at a moment's notice. Churning of coverage is endemic in the ACA's marketplace—43 percent of returning consumers to the federal on-line exchange, healthcare.gov, switched plans in 2015, often forcing change of physicians and available hospitals. [3] Those shopping for coverage in 2017 have found insurance directories even more flawed than in previous years, as more insurers exit many markets. Some physicians listed in the directories are not accepting new patients while others are not in the insurers' networks. [4] Waiting times can be very lengthy even if physicians agree to see new patients. The ACA's accountable care organizations have not saved money, and also frequently limit patients' access and continuity of care.

The insurance industry is returning to the managed care era of the 1990s, with all the increasingly built-in restrictions of choice that led to a major consumer backlash then. A recent analysis of offerings in 18 states and the District of Columbia found that 75 percent of the plans on the ACA's exchanges in 2017 will be HMOs or EPOs (exclusive provider organizations), with narrow networks that sometimes include only one large hospital system and its affiliated facilities and physicians. [5]

2. Inadequate primary care base

With the serious shortage of primary care physicians today and the near-disappearance of solo and small group practice, it has become exceptional for a patient and family to have and keep a primary care physician who knows them. More than 60 percent of U.S. physicians today are employed by others, most commonly by expanding hospital systems. Less than 10 percent of medical school graduates enter family medicine today, the broadest of the primary care specialties, with the majority of internists and pediatricians leaving primary care for subspecialties. The vacuum in primary care has led to the proliferation of urgent care centers for first-contact care, typically staffed by nurse practitioners and physician assistants, but without comprehensiveness, coordination, or continuity of care. Despite the urgency of the primary care shortage, there is still no effective national physician workforce plan on the horizon that can start to rebuild our primary care capacity.

3. Tens of millions uninsured and underinsured

As we saw in Chapter 7, there are still about 28 million Americans without health insurance, even after seven years with the ACA. That number includes 5.9 million uninsured mothers, one in five of whom are likely to have the greatest physical and mental health care needs. [6] The 19 states that refused to expand Medicaid have left 4.8 million people in a "Medicaid coverage gap" ineligible to participate in the ACA's health insurance exchanges because of incomes too low to qualify for the ACA but still above Medicaid eligibility levels. Many states impose premiums for patients on Medicaid and the Children's Health Insurance Program (CHIP), and national surveys have found that these premiums often cause recipients to dis-enroll from these programs. [7] Beyond the uninsured, there is an increasing epidemic of *underinsurance,* with 31 million people with insurance finding themselves without coverage when they need it in spite of paying more every year for premiums, deductibles, co-payments, coinsurance, and out-of-pocket costs. Figure 20.2 shows how more than two of five underinsured adults cannot afford to seek needed care. [8]

FIGURE 20.2

MORE THAN TWO OF FIVE ADULTS WHO ARE UN-DERINSURED REPORTED PROBLEMS GETTING NEEDED HEALTH CARE BECAUSE OF COSTS

Percent adults ages 19–64

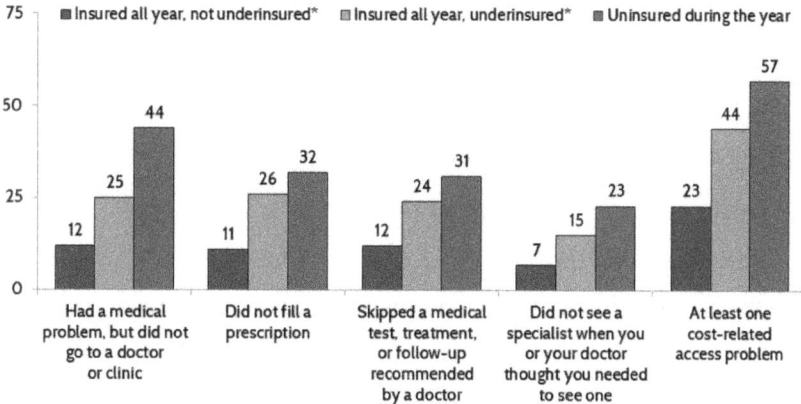

Source: The Commonwealth Fund Biennial Health Insurance Survey (2014) Reprinted
   with permission.

4. Uncontrolled costs and unaffordability

Despite the ACA, health care costs keep going up at uncon-trolled rates for American families and employers. In a system with no significant price controls, individuals and families face increas-ing costs of insurance, higher deductibles, copayments, coinsur-ance, and out-of-pocket expenses. If they have employer-sponsored insurance, they end up with higher cost-sharing as well, if their em-ployers decide to continue that coverage. Even insured, one-third of families receive additional surprise bills for services they thought would be covered. [9] An independent national poll by the Monmouth University Polling Institute in early February 2017 found that 25 percent of Americans rank health care costs as their top concern, way above job security and unemployment at 14 percent. [10]

Steven Brill, attorney, journalist, and author of *America's Bitter Pill: Money, Politics, Backroom Deals, and the Fight to Fix Our Broken Healthcare System,* was charged $197,000 for eight days in the hospital for treatment of an aortic aneurism; the CEO of his insurance company could not explain the bills to him. Brill comments about the failure of the ACA to contain health care costs:

> *It's about money: Healthcare is America's largest industry by far, employing a sixth of the country's workforce. And it is the average American family's largest single expense, whether paid out of their pockets or through taxes and insurance premiums. . . . In a country that treasures the marketplace . . . how much taming can we do when the healthcare industry spends four times as much on lobbying as the number two Beltway spender, the much-feared military-industrial complex.*[11]

As we saw in Chapter 6, many people with health insurance can no longer afford health care now that the combined annual cost of insurance and actual health care has reached about $25,000 for a typical family of four. Many patients forgo or delay necessary care, leading to worse outcomes later on when they finally get care. The staggering costs of cancer care show us how out of reach and inhumane our system has become. A one-year cost of cancer drugs often exceeds $200,000,[12] and many patients have to choose between bankruptcy and treatment.[13]

In 2014, only 11 percent of adults ages 65 and older had private long-term care insurance. Those needing nursing home care in a semi-private room face bills of about $80,000 a year, while the median cost of home care is about $20 per hour.[14] Private insurance typically does not cover these services, Medicare usually does not, and Medicaid covers only those with severe long-term service needs and supports who have spent down almost all their assets.[15]

5. Corporate profit-taking and greed at patients' expense

Not only do we have a massive medical-industrial complex, we also have a medical arms race among larger and larger corporate stakeholders in the system. This competition is mostly about making maximal profits with a predominant focus on bottom-line revenues. One example of this involves proton beam therapy for some kinds of cancer. These machines cost more than $200 million to acquire and install, so that the pressure is on to over-utilize them, whether or not they give patients longer survival (still not proven). [16] In the drive for profits, almost one-third of health care services are unnecessary, inappropriate, with some even harmful. [17] For-profit emergency rooms and urgent care centers are popping up all over the country, with this trend extending into other parts of the health care system. Two examples: for-profit behavioral health care, especially substance abuse treatment, is growing and consolidating rapidly as it attracts more investors [18]; for-profit substance abuse treatment facilities have been found to underserve vulnerable populations [19]. The rapid growth of end-of-life care through hospice gives us another example of this trend. It is now a $17 billion industry, with most hospices for-profit, but they compare poorly with their not-for-profit counterparts, spending less on nursing per patient, high rates of patients dropping out, and worse quality of care. [20]

6. A failed private health insurance industry

The private health insurance industry is on a death march, kept alive mainly by government subsidies and the generous provisions of the ACA. Insurers are finding that their enrollees are sicker than they expected and costing them more, so they raise their premiums.[21] In 2016, as examples, the largest health insurer in Texas was seeking premium increases of 59 percent [22], while the biggest plan in Tennessee would see premiums soar by an average of 62 percent.[23] Premiums in Minnesota were going up by 59 percent while rates were rising by an astounding 116 percent in Arizona. [24]

Despite the ACA, insurers continue to find ways to discriminate against the sick, such as avoiding coverage of HIV patients by offering little or no coverage of HIV drugs. [25] Humana Inc., in the process of attempting to merge with Aetna, Inc, has fallen from a four stars or higher Medicare rating of 78 percent of its plans in 2015 to just 37 percent in 2016. [26]

Many insurers are threatening or planning to leave markets in 2017, claiming insufficient profits and high expenses of coverage. Humana plans to exit Obamacare exchanges in all but a few states in 2017, citing losses of almost $1 billion. [27] UnitedHealth Group and Aetna are also planning to cut back sharply from the 2017 exchanges, [28] despite UnitedHealth Group's net earnings having gone up 23 percent on an annual basis. [29] As this trend continues, severe limits are placed on options available to consumers through the ACA's exchanges. In 2017, more than 1,000 counties in 26 states have just one health insurer available. [30]

Meanwhile, cost sharing with employees in employer-sponsored plans is going up more rapidly all the time, even as these plans carry higher deductibles; over the last ten years, these deductibles have risen by 255 percent. [31] In an attempt to ease financial insecurity, more employers are offering critical illness policies, such as one-time lump payments ranging from $5,000 to $100,000 for cancer, a heart attack, or a stroke; the cost of these policies varies widely by age, becoming prohibitive beyond the mid-50s. [32]

Former insurance industry insider Wendell Potter sums up the situation this way concerning the future of private health insurance:

> *Folks, we are guilty of magical thinking. We've fallen for insurers' deception and misdirection, hook, line and sinker. And many of us can't be persuaded that we are being duped. Meanwhile, the shareholders of the big for-profits are laughing all the way to the bank. Every single day.* [33]

7. Unacceptable quality of care

We know that insurance coverage has a lot to do with access and quality of care that is received, as well as outcomes. A 2012 estimate by the Centers for Disease Control and Prevention (CDC) estimated that 45,000 Americans were dying each year for lack of health insurance. [34] Even with private health insurance, one-third of high-need patients—defined as forgoing or delaying needed medical care or prescription medication in the last year—had unmet needs. [35] One out of three Americans lack dental insurance, leading many to forgo necessary care and to incur later preventable disease. [36] More than 31 million children in the U.S. live under, at, or near the federal poverty level; the American Academy of Pediatrics calls poverty the most serious chronic disease that children have, often leading to stunted cognitive development, impaired immune function, and psychiatric disorders. [37]

There are unacceptable big differences in the quality of care from one hospital to another across the country. A recent study that looked at some 22 million hospital admissions found that patients are three times more likely to die in the worst hospitals, with 13 times more medical complications, compared to the best hospitals. [38]

Medical errors account for about 250,000 deaths a year. [39] A recent two-year study by the ECRI Institute, a non-profit research group that studies patient safety, found that more than 7,600 so-called wrong-patient errors occurred at 181 health care organizations between 2013 and 2015. Most of these errors were caught before patients were harmed, but some were fatal, such as one patient who was not resuscitated because of being confused with another patient who had a do-not-resuscitate order on file. [40]

Adverse drug reactions are among the leading causes of hospitalization and death in the U.S., largely because of the fragmentation, discontinuity and lack of coordination of care. Patients living in areas of the country with a shortage of primary care physicians and a surplus of other specialties have more expensive care, lower quality, and worse outcomes of care, as has been shown for colorectal cancer. [41]

Despite some improvements in access through the ACA, especially with some expansion of Medicaid, disparities in health care remain widespread across the U.S. A 2013 report from the Institute of Medicine made this important point, but today's measures for quality of care still do not take socioeconomic factors into account.

> *Adverse social and economic conditions also matter greatly to health and affect a large segment of the U.S. population. Despite its large and powerful economy, the United States has higher rates of poverty and income inequality than most high-income countries. U.S. children are more likely than children in peer countries to grow up in poverty, and the proportion of today's children who will improve their socioeconomic position and earn more than their parents is smaller than in many other high-income countries. . . Finally, Americans have less access to the kinds of 'safety net' programs that help buffer the effects of adverse economic and social conditions in other countries.*[42]

8. Inadequate safety net

In my 2005 book, *Falling Through the Safety Net: Americans Without Health Insurance*, I described problems of access and affordability of care, volatility of public and private insurance coverage, and how tattered our supposed safety net was. Unfortunately, eleven years later, despite some marginal improvements under the ACA, the "safety net" continues to be porous. There continues to be a prevailing myth that everyone gets care somehow—through an extensive safety net of community health centers, emergency rooms, urgent care centers, outpatient clinics of public and private hospitals—but this is untrue for many Americans. Here are some current markers that illustrate how unreliable our safety net really is:

- Nationally, because of low Medicaid reimbursement—about 61 percent of what insurers pay for private coverage—only two-thirds of primary care physicians will see new patients on Medicaid. [43]

- The Oklahoma State Medical Association recently voted unanimously to urge physicians to leave Medicaid because of a 25 percent rate cut. [44]

- There is continuing churning of health insurance coverage from year to year under the ACA, with changing networks that often disrupt continuity of care and force patients to look again for new coverage and physicians.

- States that refused to expand Medicaid under the ACA left many patients without any coverage; a recent study estimated that at least 7,100 people will die for lack of this coverage. [45]

- Thousands of patients in South Dakota with severe diabetes, blindness, or mental illness have few alternatives for treatment, and end up warehoused unnecessarily in sterile, highly restrictive group homes, a violation of their civil liberties according to the Justice Department. [46]

- Faced with costs of curative drugs for hepatitis C up to more than $90,000 for a course of treatment, many prisons are rationing care to only the sickest of thousands of infected inmates. [47]

Larry Churchill, Ph.D., an ethicist at the University of Notre Dame, brings us this perspective:

A health system which neglects the poor and disenfranchised impoverishes the social order of which we are constituted. In a real (and not just hortatory) sense, a health care system is no better than the least well-served of its members. [48]

9. Massive, inefficient bureaucracy

The U.S. health care system is by far the most bureaucratic and expensive system in the world. Administrators in various parts of the system have grown by 3,000 percent since 1970, more than 30 times the growth in numbers of physicians. Daily interactions between the private health insurance industry, health professionals, hospitals and other facilities consume increasing amounts of time that could otherwise be spent on patient care if we had a simplified single-payer financing system. These markers illustrate the extent of our administrative morass:

- U.S. nurses spend more than 13 hours per week to obtain prior authorizations for services, compared to none in Canada. [49]
- Hospital administrative costs in the U.S. account for more than 25 percent of total hospital expenditures, more than double those in Scotland and Canada, both single-payer countries. [50]
- There is an ongoing large administrative burden for the ACA's exchanges to determine eligibility for qualified health plans and subsidies/tax credits, especially in verifying annual income and family size, which are subject to change from year to year. [51]
- IRS forms used by employers, insurers and exchanges are extremely complex; as examples, instructions for forms 1094-C and 1095-C, used by large employers with more than 50 full-time or full-time equivalent employees, fill 13 pages with dense, two column print. [52]
- CMS projects that more than $2.7 trillion will be spent for private health insurance overhead and administration of government programs (mostly Medicare and Medicaid) between 2014

and 2022, including $273.6 billion in *new* administrative costs attributable to the ACA's expanded Medicaid program. [53]

- Cybercriminals have found stolen health records to be profitable; more than 100 million health care records were compromised in 2015 alone, including from such large insurers as Anthem Inc. and Primera Blue Cross. [54]

The health insurance overhead in the U.S. is $792 per capita, far higher than five comparison countries, as shown in Figure 20.3.

Timothy Jost, J.D., professor emeritus of law at the Washington and Lee University School of Law and a leading expert on health care law, observes:

We are doomed to continue to struggle with this complexity as long as we stubbornly cling to a private health insurance-based health care financing system. [55]

FIGURE 20.3

INSURANCE OVERHEAD IN 6 COUNTRIES

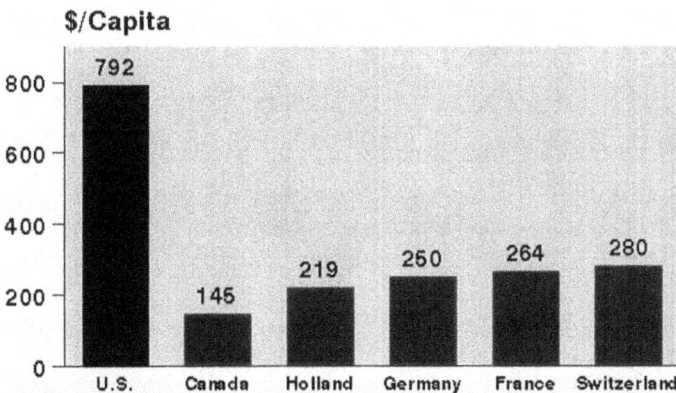

Source: OECD, 2016; NCHS; CIHI

Note: Figures adjusted for Purchasing Power Parity; data are for 2016 or most recent available

10. Squandered public taxpayer money on exploitive private plans

As we saw in Chapters 1 and 2, corporatization and consoli-dation have been dominant trends in U.S. health care, especially over the last 25 years. Most people assume that we have a mostly private system with little government involvement except for such programs as Medicare and Medicaid. But privatization of Medicare and Medicaid has also been increasing rapidly, together with subsi-dization of the private health insurance industry over many years, accelerated by the ACA since 2010. Most people find it surprising to believe that the government is already paying for almost two-thirds of U.S. health care spending—about $1.9 trillion in 2013, much of that subsidizing private health care industries, especially private health insurance. [56] Yet we still have major increasing problems of access, cost, affordability, and equity in our system, although there is more than enough money in the system to provide universal ac-cess through a single-payer system for all Americans.

The big problem is that the public purse is being exploited for the private gain of corporate stakeholders in the system, and their economic and political power has thwarted meaningful reform for many years. It is already obvious that our deregulated marketplace is not sustainable. One of the consequences is that we can no longer afford to fund necessary care for many people, as illustrated by the growing public health threat of hepatitis C. There are now 3.2 mil-lion Americans with the chronic hepatitis C virus, the leading cause of liver-related deaths, hepatocellular carcinoma, and liver trans-plant. It can be cured with the latest drugs that cost about $100,000 for a full course of treatment over a year. [57] But most are uninsured or underinsured, and many are in prison. So who will pay for this treatment at a time of budget cuts of federal and state safety net pro-grams and with no regulation of drug prices?

11. Increasing burnout of health professionals with limited professional and clinical autonomy

As described in Chapter 13, burnout rates for U.S. physicians are increasing rapidly, especially in the primary care specialties confronted by the frustrations of our current system and increasing dissatisfaction with their practice environment. Electronic medical records, while intended to improve patient care, are used more for billing purposes, leading about one-third of their physician users to increasing frustration and burnout. [58] Almost one-half of U.S. physicians are experiencing some symptoms of burnout, while other health professionals, especially nurses and receptionists, are also dealing with burnout more often than in the past.

For some years, the Triple Aim has been a goal for improving the quality of health care in this country—by enhancing the patient experience, improving population health, and reducing costs. An important recent article defines the problem and proposes a fourth aim—care of the patient requires care of the provider, together with practical steps to address that goal. [59]

12. Politicized health policy vs. evidence-based science

So many issues related to health care in this country have become politicized without connection to information or experience, and used as political weapons seeking narrow interests of their proponents. We have seen how Republicans have been insistent in their opposition to the Affordable Care Act, and how 20 states turned down federal money to expand Medicaid to meet real unmet needs in their states. Another example of politicized health policy without grounding in evidence or medical need is the widespread opposition to women's reproductive rights, as illustrated by defunding of Planned Parenthood in many states, ranging from Texas, Arkansas, Alabama, and North Carolina in the South to Utah, Kansas, Wisconsin, Ohio and New Hampshire. [60] These are extreme and harmful policies, typically targeted against abortion clinics (only 1 percent of Planned Parenthood's services) but cutting millions of women off from such other essential services as contraceptive care, cancer screenings, and other vital services. Some states go so far as to make abortion unavailable even in the case of rape or incest.

In their recent book, *It's Even Worse Than It Was: How the American Constitutional System Collided with the New Politics of Extremism,* Thomas E. Mann and Norman J. Ornstein describe the deep dysfunction of American politics today:

> *The main problem remains an insurgent outlier Republican Party, in the midst of an existential struggle for its soul. A very conservative but somewhat pragmatic wing is facing, and losing to, a group of radicals who yearn not for a smaller but efficient government but for a society largely free of government. Equally dangerous, the radicals have been able, at the state level, to implement a sharply more intrusive role of government in areas where they welcome it, like abortion and contraception.* [61]

Concluding comment:

The above health care landscape is not a good picture. It is primarily a confrontation between profit-seeking corporate stakeholders and the common good, still based on the notion that free markets can fix our health care problems. It is long overdue to put this discredited claim to rest.

In their recent book, *American Amnesia: How the War on Government Led Us to Forget What Made America Prosper*, Jacob B. Hacker and Paul Pierson, professors of political science at Yale University and the University of California Berkeley, respectively, give us this helpful insight:

If we take on the robber barons of health care, finance, energy, and other sectors, we can generate even bigger benefits—from slower growth of health spending to lower pollution, from longer lives to stronger financial security, from increased educational opportunity to decreased economic hardship. . . . There is money on the table just waiting to be picked up. . . . We can make our already prosperous society much more prosperous. And in doing so, we can also get our troubled democracy back on track. [62]

In the next chapter, we will consider what lessons can be learned from this sixty-year transformation of U.S. health care.

Endnotes:

1. Davis, K Stremikis, K, Squires, D et al. *Mirror, Mirror on the Wall, 2014 update: How the U.S. Health Care System Compares Internationally.* The Commonwealth Fund, June 16, 2014.

2. Johnson, CY. Health-care sign-ups fall far short of forecasts. *The Washington Post,* August 27, 2016.

3. Rau, J. Frustration runs deep for customers forced to change marketplace plans routinely. *Kaiser Health News,* October 17, 2016.

4. Mathews, AW. Insurers' offerings dwindle. *Wall Street Journal,* September 1, 2016: B1.

5. Hancock, J. Insurers' flawed directories leave patients scrambling for in-network doctors. *Kaiser Health News,* December 5, 2016.

6. Karpman, M, Gates, J, Kenney, GM et al. How are moms faring under the Affordable Care Act? Evidence through 2014. Urban Institute, May 5, 2016.

7. Saloner, B, Hochhalter, W, Sabik, L. Medicaid and CHIP premiums and access to care: A systematic review. *Pediatrics* 137 (3), March 2016.

8. Issue Brief. The problem of underinsurance and how rising deductibles will make it worse. Findings from the Commonwealth Fund Biennial Health Insurance Survey, 2014. The Commonwealth Fund, May 20, 2015.

9. Edwards, HS. You only think you're covered. *Time*, March 14, 2016. Brill, S. *America's Bitter Pill: Money, Politics, Backroom Deals, and the Fight to Fix Our Broken Healthcare System.* New York. *Random House.* 2015, pp. 7-8.

10. Health care is top concern of American families. 3-in-10 struggling to maintain current financial situation. *Monmouth University Polling Institute*, February 7, 2017.

11. Brill, S. *America's Bitter Pill: Money, Politics, Back Room Deals, and the Fight to Fix Our Broken Healthcare System,* New York. *Random House.* 2015, pp.7-8

12. Langreth, R, Koons C. The cancer doctor is leading the attack on astronomical drug prices. *Bloomberg Business*, June 1, 2015.

13. Reinberg, S. Cancer's financial burden tied to poorer survival, study finds. *U.S. News & World Report*, January 26, 2016.

14. Genworth. 2015. Genworth 2015 Cost of Care Survey. Richmond, VA: Genworth Financial Inc.

15. Johnson, RW. Who is covered by private long-term care insurance? *Urban Institute*, August 2, 2016.

16. Gold, J. Proton beam therapy heats up hospital arms race. *Kaiser Health News*, May 31, 2013.

17. Caper, P. The ills of money-driven medicine. Op-Ed, *Bangor Daily News*, May 21, 2012.

18. Kutscher, B. Coverage parity draws investors to behavioral health. *Modern Healthcare*, July 20, 2015.

19. Cummings, JR, Wen, H, Ko, M. Decline in public substance abuse disorder treatment centers most serious in counties with high shares of black residents. *Health Affairs*, June 2016.

20. Whoriskey, P, Keating, D. Dying and profits: The evolution of hospice. *The Washington Post*, December 26, 2014.

21. Pear, R. Newest policyholders under health law are sicker and costlier to insurers. *New York Times,* March 30, 2016.

22. Associated Press. Insurance rates going up: New concerns for Obamacare. *New York Times*, June 2, 2016.

23. Radnofsky, L, Armour, S. States approve steep health-premium increases. *Wall Street Journal,* August 24, 2016.

24. Montgomery, D. Minnesota's health insurance premium hike is fourth-highest in nation. *Pioneer Press*, October 24, 2016.

25. Andrews, M. 7 insurers alleged to use skimpy drug coverage to discourage HIV patients. *Kaiser Health News*, October 18, 2016.

26. Darie, T. Humana drops after ratings for its Medicare plans decline. *Bloomberg News*, October 12, 2016.

27. Ferris, S. Humana to leave 'substantially all' ObamaCare markets. *The Hill*, July 21, 2016.

28. Mathews, AW. Aetna backs off plans to expand its ACA business. *Wall Street Journal*, August 3, 2016.

29. Herman, B. UnitedHealth Group's earnings soar as ACA retreat ramps up. *Modern Healthcare*, October 18, 2016.

30 Associated Press. Lack of choice in health insurance markets a growing problem, October 28, 2016.

31. Woolhandler, D, Himmelstein, DU. Healthcare inequality on the rise. *The Hill*, August 2, 2016.

32. Bernard, TS. Insurance for critical illness may add security, but at a cost. *New York Times*, March 18, 2016.

33. Potter, W. It's way past time for us to stop deluding ourselves about private health insurers. *The Progressive Populist*, p. 20.: September 1, 2016:

34. CDC reports 45,000 Americans die each year for lack of health insurance. *Daily Kos*, October 15, 2012.

35. Salzberg, CAS, Hayes, SL, McCarthy, DC et al. Health system performance for the high-need patient: A look at access to care and patient care experiences. New York. *The Commonwealth Fund*, August 29, 2016.

36. Potter, W. America's silent epidemic will end when public officials stop kowtowing to a single special interest. *Huffington Post*, June 2, 2016.

37. Healy, M. Doctors group calls on pediatricians to address child poverty. *Los Angeles Times*, March 9, 2016.

38. Abelson, R. Go to the wrong hospital and you're 3 times more likely to die. *New York Times*, December 14, 2016.

39. Bakalar, N. Medical errors may cause over 250,000 deaths a year. *New York Times*, May 3, 2016.

40. Beck, M. Wrong-patient errors called common. Wall Street Journal, September 26, 2016: A 2.

41. Roetzheim, RG, Pal, N, Gonzalez, EC et al. The effects of physician supply on the early detection of colorectal cancer. *J Fam Pract* 48 (11): 850-858, 1999.

42. Woolf, SH, Aron, L, eds. U.S. Health in International Perspective: Shorter Lives, Poorer Health. National Research Council. Institute of Medicine. Washington, D.C., the *National Academies Press*, 2013.

43. Decker, SL. Two-thirds of primary care physicians accepted new Medicaid patients in 2011-2012: A baseline to measure future acceptance rates. *Health Affairs* 32 (7): 1183-1187, 2013.

44. Hoberock, B. Oklahoma State Medical Association urges doctors to mull leaving Medicaid over 25 percent rate cut. *Tulsa World*, April 1, 2016.

45. Dickman, SL, Himmelstein, DU, McCormick, D et al. Health and financial harms of 25 states' decision to opt out of Medicaid. *Health Affairs Blog*, January 30, 2014.

46. Apuzzo, M. South Dakota wrongly puts thousands in nursing homes, government says. *New York Times*, May 2, 2016.

47. Loftus, P, Fields, G. Costly drugs for prisoners with on public budgets. *Wall Street Journal*, September 13, 2016: A1.

48. Churchill, LR. *Rationing Health Care in America: Perceptions and Principles of Justice.* Notre Dame, Ind; University of Notre Dame, 1987: 103.

49. Morra, D, Nicholson, S, Levinson, W et al. U.S. physician practices versus Canadians: spending nearly four times as much money interacting with payers. *Health Affairs* 30 (8): 1443-1450, 2011.

50. Himmelstein, DU, Mun, M, Bisse, R et al. A comparison of hospital administrative costs in eight nations: U.S. costs exceed all others by far. *Health Affairs*, September 2014.

51. Office of the Inspector General. Not all of the federally facilitated marketplace's internal controls were effective in ensuring that individuals were properly determined eligible for qualified health plans and insurance affordability programs. Department of Health and Human Services. Washington, D.C., August 2015.

52. Jost, T. Implementing health reform: Tax form instructions. *Health Affairs Blog*, August 29, 2014.

53. Himmelstein, DU, Woolhandler, S. The post-launch problem: The Affordable Care Act's persistently high administrative costs. *Health Affairs Blog*, May 27, 2015.

54. Woodward, C. Health files make for a juicy target for thieves. *Boston Globe online*, August 7, 2016.

55. Jost, T. As quoted by McCanne, D. Quote of the Day online. Instruction sheets for completing ACA tax forms—a proxy for ACA complexity. August 29, 2014.

56. Himmelstein, DU, Woolhandler, S. The current and projected taxpayer shares of U.S. health costs. *Amer J Public Health* online, January 21, 2016.

57. Chahal, HS, Marseille, EA, Tice, JA et al. Cost-effectiveness of early treatment of hepatitis C virus genotype 1 by stage of liver fibrosis in a U.S. treatment-naïve population. *JAMA Internal Medicine* online, November 23, 2015.

58. Doyle, K. Doctors less satisfied, more burned out with electronic records. *Reuters*, June 28, 2016.

59. Bodenheimer, T, Simsky, C. From triple to quadruple aim: Care of the patient requires care of the provider. *Ann Fam Med* 12 (6): 573-576, 2014.

60. Where the GOP defunded Planned Parenthood. *Emily's List*, April 18, 2016.

61. Mann, TE, Ornstein, NJ. *It's Even Worse Than It Looks: How the American Constitutional System Collided with the New Politics of Extremism.* New York. *Basic Books*, 2016, p. 204.

62. Hacker, JS, Pierson, P. *American Amnesia: How the War on Government Led Us to Forget What Made America Prosper.* New York. *Simon & Schuster*, 2016, p. 338.

CHAPTER 21

WHAT CAN WE LEARN FROM THIS DYSFUNCTIONAL EVOLUTION OF HEALTH CARE?

A much freer market in health care and health insurance can work, can deliver high quality, technically innovative care at much lower cost, and solve the pathologies of the pre-existing system.

> —John H. Cochrane, senior fellow of the Hoover Institution and adjunct scholar of the Cato Institute [1]

We've engaged in a massive and failed experiment in market-based medicine in the U.S. Rhetoric about the benefits of competition and profit-driven health care can no longer hide the reality: Our health system is in shambles.

> —Marcia Angell, M.D., former editor of *The New England Journal of Medicine* and author of *The Truth About Drug Companies: How They Deceive Us and What We Can Do About It.* [2]

The above opposing views of health care in America cut to the heart of the fundamental systemic situation creating and perpetuating our problems in health care, especially the role of markets vs. the government and how to finance health care. Before we review the lessons we have learned over the last 60 years in U.S. health care, let's look at the larger picture of politics over that period, since health care is just one part of our overall economy.

In his new book, *How Did We Get Into This Mess?: Politics, Equality, Nature,* George Monbiot shows us how neoliberalism has been *the* defining ideology of our times. As he writes:

> So pervasive has neoliberalism become that we seldom even recognize it as an ideology. We appear to accept the neoliberal proposition that this utopian, millenarian faith (which holds that the free market, unimpeded by government intervention, will answer all human needs) is nothing more than a description of a neutral, natural force—a kind of biological law, like Darwin's theory of evolution. [3]

James K. Galbraith, leading economist of our time, further observed in 2015:

> Neoliberalism is mainly about transferring public assets into private hands. So, under neoliberalism, we have seen not only a rollback of social programs and the additional liberalization of the labor market which includes an orchestrated assault on labor unions by corporate interests and the economic elite, but increasing valuation of asset income, which spearheads economic inequality. . . . The top 3 percent hold over double the wealth held by America's poorest 90 percent of the population. [4]

Takeaway Lessons from the Transformation of U.S. Health Care

1. Market failure

Our experiment with market-based medicine, going back some 40 years, has been a failure, except for enriching corporate stakeholders in the medical-industrial complex. Most economists have believed that health care markets work like other markets, where competition can keep down prices and patients can shop for the best deal. That belief, however, has been thoroughly discredited over the years for many reasons: patients don't really know their needs, urgency of time is often a factor, information is not transparent, there is asymmetry between physicians' and patients' knowledge, and so on. The theory that patients can save themselves and the health care system money by becoming savvier shoppers was rebutted by a recent study that found that less than 7 percent of total health care spending in 2011 was paid by consumers for "shoppable" services.[5] Beyond these and other reasons, our experience over the last three decades has proven that supposed "competition" in health care markets has *not* controlled prices or costs.

Some economists saw this problem from the beginning. Dr. Friedrich A. Hayek, leading economist from the last century, professor of social and moral sciences at the University of Chicago from 1950 to 1962, predicted the downsides of market capitalism in 1946:

> *Market capitalism will have the same inefficient, exploitive outcome as Soviet Communism if the ownership of resources becomes concentrated in the hands of fewer and fewer large corporations, and if economic business decisions come to be made by those relatively few individuals who own and/or operate large concentrated corporations.*[6]

Kenneth Arrow, a leading economist at Columbia University, observed back in 1963 that uncertainty would be the root cause of market failure in health care, both for patients and physicians dealing with the unavoidable uncertainties as to diagnosis, treatment, and prognosis of illness. [7] Insurers have dealt with uncertainty by experience rating and medical underwriting and by avoiding, if they can, sicker patients.

There is much less competition in health care than market enthusiasts claim (though the belief in market competition remains a standard part of the rhetoric of virtually all Republican politicians!). Instead, accelerated by the ACA, we have increasing consolidation of hospital systems and insurers, with wide latitude to set prices to what the traffic will bear. Yet many economists still cling to the myth of competitive health care markets, as illustrated by this response to the soaring prices of oral cancer drugs by Mark V. Pauly, Ph.D. He has heralded the concept of moral hazard for years, whereby he claims that patients are prone to irresponsibly seek out and overuse health care services. [8] His preposterous "solution" to the problem of high drug costs:

> *If we consumers want to do something about rising prices for cancer drugs, we need (according to the hardhearted economist) to do what happens when prices for gas, or steak, or designer ties is rising—we need to walk away from them. A tepid demand response will itself temper prices as well as total spending, and perhaps offer a cautionary lesson for future health care price increases.* [9]

2. Consumer directed health care another failure.

Another long-held belief that needs to go away is the concept of consumer-driven health care (CDHC)—the idea that "empowered" patients in an "ownership society" will contain health care costs by becoming more prudent about their decisions to seek care. What that really means is that patients have to have "more skin in the game" by larger deductibles, co-payments, and other restrictions. CDHC has been the underlying principle for conventional health insurance for many years, despite growing evidence that the more cost-sharing with patients, the worse their outcomes as they forgo or delay necessary care. In effect, CDHC enables the growing shift of responsibility for health care costs from employers, insurers, and federal/state governments to patients. (10)

We should have learned by now that higher deductibles do not constrain health care costs, both because of experience over many years and because of a persistent fact—only about 20 percent of people account for 80 percent of health care costs. The 20 percent needing health care for major illness or accidents blow through their deductibles quickly, after which there is no cost containment. Meanwhile, the tradeoff of high deductibles in everyday use is to sacrifice access to care and create financial hardships leading patients to forgo necessary care and have worse outcomes. We have to recognize that the main purpose of higher deductibles is to reduce spending in health care by insurers, employers and government plans, not to help patients. [11]

Drs. Woolhandler and Himmelstein give us an international view of the results of cost-sharing for cost-control:

> *International evidence indicates that cost-sharing is neither necessary nor particularly effective for cost-control; the U.S. has high cost-sharing and the highest costs. Canada, which outlawed copayments and deductibles in 1981, has seen both faster health improvement and slower cost growth.[12] Canadian provinces control costs by tax-based funding; global hospital budgeting; binding, negotiated physician fee schedules; and a simple unified single-payer structure that minimized administrative burdens and costs. Scotland, which has eschewed market-based policies and patient payments—even going so far as to abolish parking fees—has costs about half those in the U.S. Scots view patients as owners of their health care system, not its customers.[13]*

3. Private health insurance is a major problem, is obsolete, and should be abandoned.

The private health insurance industry has had a long run, is antithetical to reform, and continues to game the system at the expense of patients and taxpayers. Even after the ACA, it still discriminates against the sick, by such means as benefit designs that limit access, high cost-sharing, inadequate provider networks, restrictive drug formularies, and deceptive marketing practices. It consumes 15 to 20 percent of the health care dollar in bureaucracy, administrative overhead, and profits, plus receiving large subsidies from the government. Its products have become unaffordable to millions of people even as its benefits have continued to decrease in an increasing segmented market.

It has become difficult, even impossible, for patients with cancer to gain in-network coverage at leading cancer centers. [14] Meanwhile, insurers are marketing new kinds of inadequate gap insurance, or "insurance on insurance." These supplemental plans are exempt from the ACA's requirements, and include coverage for high deductibles and copays for treatment and lump sum payments upon diagnosis of such conditions as cancer, heart disease and stroke. [15]

Insurers leave the market whenever their profits fall below expectations of their CEOs and shareholders. At the end of 2016, at least 1.4 million people in 32 states lost their ACA coverage when insurers exited their markets, leaving them fewer choices than earlier. In North Carolina, as an example, Blue Cross Blue Shield became the only insurer in 95 of the state's 100 counties. [16] Medical out-of-pocket costs now drag more than 11 million insured people into poverty as deductibles, copays, and co-insurance rates continue to climb. [17]

Segmented risk pools are the antithesis of what we need, as Dr. Henry Sigerist, Director of the Institute of the History of Medicine at the Johns Hopkins University, recognized as far back as 1944:

> *Illness is an unpredictable risk for the individual family, but we know fairly accurately how much illness a large group of people will have, how much medical care they will require, and how many days they will have to spend in hospitals. In other words, we cannot budget the cost of illness for the individual family but we can budget it for the nation. The principle must be to spread the risk among as many people as possible . . . The experience of the last 15 years in the United States [since 1931] has, in my opinion, demonstrated that voluntary health insurance does not solve the problem of the nation. It reaches only certain groups and is always at the mercy of economic fluctuations . . . Hence, if we decide to finance medical services through insurance, the insurance system must be compulsory.* [18]

Gerald Friedman, Ph.D., professor of economics at the University of Massachusetts and author of the classic 2013 study on the costs of single-payer national health insurance, [19] brings us this important insight:

> *In many commodity markets, profits are a reward for making good products at low cost. Profits reward the company that makes my laptop, for example, giving it an incentive to produce a quality computer at low price; the more they sell, the more they profit. The incentives in health care are different, however. Rather than increasing sales, health insurers profit by screening customers, segmenting*

the market so as to exclude those likely to use health care ("lemon dropping") while attracting the healthy and lucky who use less health care ("cherry picking"). While profitable, such activities add to the cost of America's bloated health care administration, raising a question that we should ask of all health care insurers: how many patients did your company help today? [20]

4. Not enough regulation in present system

Although we are being assured constantly by market enthusiasts that competition and less regulation will somehow solve our health care problems, we know from long experience that this is a myth. Here are some examples among many of how lax the ACA has been on the health insurance industry: [21]

- Most regulatory authority is given to the states, many of which were hostile to the ACA and where the insurance lobby dominates state capitols; the federal government cannot deny premium rate increases of 10 percent or more.
- The Center for Public Integrity has found that one-half of state insurance commissioners who have left their jobs in the last ten years have gone to work for the industry they were supposedly regulating. [22]
- Oversight and regulation of insurance networks are left to the states, with minimal federal guidance—"marketplace plans must maintain a network that is sufficient in number and types of providers so that all services will be accessible without reasonable delay." [23]
- HHS was originally planning to provide network-breadth information for 35 states; the latest goal is to shrink the pilot tool to just 4 states. [24]

- The Obama administration acceded to the industry's lobbying against a requirement to report executive and employee compensation data.
- Remarkably, state insurance regulators across the country have been approving 2017 rate increases *higher* than those requested by many insurers, even with the support of Andy Slavitt, CMS's acting administrator of Medicare and Medicaid. [25]
- Insurers can accumulate surplus profits free from regulatory oversight.

The drug industry also benefits from lax regulation, for which it lobbies so effectively. One example is the recent passage by Congress of the 21st Century Cures Act, which drastically lowers the standards of FDA approval of new drugs. The previous gold standard for effectiveness depended on rigorous random-controlled trials. The new "standard" is "real world evidence," which is really uncontrolled observational data. [26]

5. *"Quality" measures have failed and are counter productive.*

The ACA introduced new "value-based" initiatives that theoretically might improve the quality of care, such as pay-for-performance (P4P) report cards for physicians and accountable care organizations. There are now more than 150 quality metrics in use for outpatient services, such as rates of screening mammography and testing for cholesterol levels. There is still no evidence, however, that these quality measures improve care. They are rudimentary, are burdensome on physicians and staff (who spend more than 15 hours per week reporting the measures at an average cost to a physician's practice of more than $40,000), and are easily gamed by physicians' employers by upcoding (exaggerating diagnoses to make them appear sicker) for maximal revenue. [27] Moreover, because these measures do not effectively provide risk adjustment for socioeconomic factors, these measures penalize safety net institutions dealing with poor and disadvantaged populations. [28] While well intended, this policy also becomes a disincentive for physicians to serve these populations because they will receive lower scores on quality measures compared to practicing in higher-income areas.

In his 2015 book, *The Health Gap: The Challenge of an Unequal World*, Sir Michael Marmot, professor of epidemiology and public health at University College London and president of the World Medical Association, calls attention to the poor health outcomes of people dealing with adverse social and economic conditions in the U.S. with higher rates of poverty and income than in most high-income countries. He also notes that Americans have less access to safety net programs than in other countries. As he reminds us:

> *When people get sick, they need access to high-quality medical care. Medical care saves lives. But it is not the lack of medical care that causes illness in the first place. Inequalities in health arise from inequalities in society. Social conditions have a determining impact on access to medical care, as they do on access to the other aspects of society that lead to good health.* [29]

6. Health care is not just another commodity, but an essential human right.

The U.S. still stands alone among advanced countries in not accepting health care as a basic human right. Stakeholders in our profit-driven system see health care as a big industry where financial bottom lines drive policy and access to care depends on patients' ability to pay. Whether we admit it or not, we are all in the same boat, regardless of our income—at some or many times in our lives we will have a serious illness or accident that can bankrupt us or diminish our futures. These two observations make the case in a compelling way that health care should not be just another commodity for sale on a free market:

> *In our society, some aspects of life are off-limits to commerce. We prohibit the selling of children and the buying of wives, juries, and kidneys. Tainted blood is an inevitable consequence of paying blood donors; even sophisticated laboratory tests cannot compensate for blood that is sold rather than given as a gift. Like blood, health care is too precious, intimate, and corruptible to entrust to the market.*
>
> — Steffie Woolhander, M.D. David Himmelstein, M.D. [30]

> *There is a moral right to health care, but not of the sort often claimed. It is a right grounded not on purchasing power, merit, or social worth, but in human need. The right to health care finds its rationale in a knowledge of common vulnerability to disease and death . . .*
>
> —Larry Churchill, Ph.D. [31]

7. Present health care policies will bankrupt patients, families, states and the federal government.

As we saw in Chapter 6, there is no cost containment of health care costs on the horizon. Six years after its passage, the ACA has failed to restrain either costs or prices. Instead, its generous provisions have fueled expanded markets throughout the medical-industrial complex at the expense of taxpayers and patients through ever increasing cost sharing. In effect, the ACA is a massive bailout of private interests profiting on the backs of sick and injured Americans.

With the costs of health insurance and care now up to about $25,000 a year for a family of four, in times of static incomes with reduced purchasing power, where will this end, even in the near term? The open market still provides about one-third more health care services than are necessary or appropriate. The budgets of state governments increasingly fall short of their residents' needs, as illustrated by the inability of meager Medicaid budgets to cover care of a growing number of patients with hepatitis C. Meanwhile, the federal government is confronted by widespread fraud in its public programs and the burden of ongoing subsidies generously granted to the insurance industry through the ACA. Given all this, we cannot avoid real accounting much longer. We will have to come to terms with the reality that the more unaffordable health care becomes, the less access to essential care Americans will have, the worse their outcomes will be, and the greater political backlash we can expect.

8. Inadequate leadership by the medical profession

As we saw in Chapter 13, most physicians today are employed by large corporate employers, especially expanding hospital systems, whether they are in clinic or hospital-based practice. They have lost much of their negotiating influence and clinical autonomy of previous generations. Their organizations have for the most part been focused on their own self-interest, thereby diminishing their leadership role toward health care reform in the public interest. Unfortunately, conflicts of interests are all too common, as illustrated by this one recent example, among many—Doctor-owned distributorships operate in 43 states, most commonly in spinal surgery, where surgeons perform almost twice as many spinal-fusion procedures compared to those not in such arrangements. [32] The traditional social contract between the medical profession and society needs to be rebuilt.

9. Extensive economic and political power of corporate stakeholders in the medical-industrial complex, with a compliant media, stand in the way of financing reform.

As shown throughout this book, the economic and political power and influence of corporate stakeholders in our health care marketplace is an obvious barrier to reform. Owned as they are by large corporate interests, the "mainstream" media take less than an objective or investigative approach to the news. Two recent examples illustrate this problem:

- Despite having supported the importation of prescription drugs during the 2008 campaign, President Obama opposed it in the ACA and appointed Dr. Robert Califf, a cardiologist opposed to regulation with deep ties to corporately-funded research, as the new head of the FDA in 2015. [33]

- Support for single-payer NHI was a key part of Bernie Sanders' presidential campaign; predictably, *The Washington Post*, sold in 2013 to libertarian Amazon CEO Jeff Bezoz, with a net worth of about $49.8 billion, ran 16 negative stories on Bernie Sanders in 16 hours. [34]

10. We need a larger role of government to advance the common good in health care.

We have to recognize that we have to change the financing system in order to change the delivery of health care for the common good. That will require a significant role of government to make that happen. In their excellent new book, Jacob Hacker and Paul Pierson, *American Amnesia: How the War on Government Led Us to Forget What Made America Prosper*, professors of political science at Yale University and the University of California Berkeley, respectively, remind us that:

It takes government—a lot of government—for advanced societies to flourish. But Americans have never been good at acknowledging government's necessary role in supporting both freedom and prosperity . . . The United States got rich because it got government more or less right. We suffer, in short from a kind of mass historical forgetting, a distinctively 'American Amnesia.' [35]

Joseph Stiglitz, Ph.D., Nobel Laureate in Economics and former chief economist at the World Bank, brings us this important insight:

Markets do not lead to efficient outcomes, let alone outcomes that comport with social justice. As a result, there is often good reason for government intervention to improve the efficiency of the market. Just as the Great Depression should have made it evident that the market does not work as well as its advocates claim, our recent Roaring

Nineties should have made it self-evident that the pursuit of self-interest does not necessarily lead to overall economic efficiency. [36]

As Theodore Marmor, Jerry Mashaw, and John Pakutka observe in their 2014 book, *Social Insurance: America's Neglected Heritage and Contested Future*:

In health care, the "invisible hand" fails to drive down costs, improve quality, or ensure distributional outcomes that are regarded as fair. We can tinker with the rules, regulations and payment schemes that govern medical care, but the forces that increase the demands for and supply of more care are relentless. Only powerful coun-

tervailing institutions can keep them under control. Only governments have the necessary authority, assuming they have the political will to use it. [37]

11. Finally, we have to admit that today's health care is unsustainable, and is in crisis that is still largely denied. But there is a fix if we look to the experience of other advanced countries around the world.

Concluding Comment

The political landscape over the last 35 years has been unfavorable for health care reform. Robert Kuttner sums up this period:

> *The era since 1981 has been one of turning away from public remediation, toward tax cuts, limited social spending, deregulation, and privatization. None of this worked well, except for the very top. For everyone else, the shift to conservative policies generated more economic insecurity.*[38]

Two big questions are still unanswered: Who is the health care system for? Is health care a human right based on medical need, or a privilege based on ability to pay?

We can see a better future in our health care, but never with the status quo. In the next chapter, we will consider three major financing alternatives to bail us out of this mess, only one of which will give us what we need.

Endnotes:

1. Cochrane, JH. What to do when Obamacare unravels. *Wall Street Journal,* December 26, 2013: A13.

2. Angell, M. Sweeping health care reform proposed by the nation's top physicians. Press release. Physicians for a National Health Program. Chicago, IL, May 1, 2001.

3. Monbiot, G. *How Did We Get Into This Mess?: Politics, Equality, Nature.* New York. *Verso,* 2016, p. 3.

4. Galbraith, JK. As quoted by Polychroniou, CJ. James K. Galbraith on the human cost of inequality in the neoliberal age. *Truthout,* November 12, 2015. Available at: htpp://www.truth-out,org/opinion/item/33622-james-k-galbraith…

5. Andrews, M. Consumer choices have limited impact on U.S. health care spending: Study. *Kaiser Health News,* March 4, 2016.

6. Hayek, FA. *American Economic Review,* 1946.

7. Arrow, KJ. Uncertainty and the welfare economics of medical care. *American Economic Review* 53: 941-973, 1963.

8. Pauly, MV. The economics of moral hazard: Comment. *American Economic Review* 58 (3), 1968.

9. Pauly, MV. Maybe we are to blame in part for rising cancer drug prices. *Philly.com,* May 9, 2016.

10. Geyman, JP. Moral hazard and consumer-driven health care: A fundamentally flawed concept. *Intl J Health Services* 37 (2): 333-346, 2007.

11. McCanne, D. Comment in Quote-of-the-Day on the November 2016 National Bureau of Economic Research report, NBER Working Paper 22802, November 7, 2016.

12. Himmelstein, DU, Woolhandler, S. Cost control in a parallel universe: Medicare spending in the United States and Canada. *Arch Intern Med* 172: 1764-1766, 2012.

13. Woolhandler, S, Himmelstein, DU. Life of debt: Underinsurance in America. *J Gen Intern Med* on line, April 25, 2013.

14. Tracer, Z, Darie, T. More than 1 million in Obamacare to lose plans as insurers quit. *Bloomberg News,* October 14, 2016.

15. Silverman, RE. For workers, an 'insurance on insurance.' *Wall Street Journal,* December 7, 2016, B5.

16. Tracer, Z, Darie, T. More than 1 million in Obamacare to lose plans as insurers quit. *Bloomberg News,* October 14, 2016.

17. Herman, B. Uninsured rate drops, but medical expenses still drag millions into poverty. *Modern Healthcare,* September 13, 2016.

18. Sigerist, HE. Medical care for all the people. *Canadian Journal of Public Health* 35 (7): 258, 1944.

19. Friedman, G. Funding H. R. 676. The Expanded and Improved Medicare for All Act. How We Can Afford a National Single Payer Health Plan. *Physicians for a National Health Program*, Chicago, Il, July 31, 2013.

20. Friedman, G. An open letter to the *New York Times* that was rejected. February 6, 2016.

21 Williams, BW. Compromised: The Affordable Care Act and Politics of Defeat. *CreateSpace Independent Publishing Platform*. North Charleston, South Carolina, 2014, 66-75.

22. Mishak, MJ. Drinks, junkets and jobs: How the insurance industry courts state commissioners. *The Washington Post*, October 2, 2016.

23. Issue Brief. Implementing the Affordable Care Act state regulation of marketplace plan provider networks. *The Commonwealth Fund*, May 5, 2015.

24. Andrews, M. How narrow is it? Gov't begins test of comparison tool for health plan networks. *Kaiser Health News*, October 14, 2016.

25. Lee, J, O'Donnell, J. Regulators approve higher health premiums to strengthen Obamacare insurers. *USA TODAY*, October 19, 2016.

26. Gaffney, A. Congress just quietly handed drug companies a dangerous victory. *New Republic*, December 14, 2016.

27. Casalino, LP, Gans, D, Weber, R et al. U.S. physician practices spend more than $15.4 billion annually to report quality measures. *Health Affairs*, March 2016.

28. Woolhandler, S, Himmelstein, DU. Pay-for-performance initiatives and safety net hospitals. *Ann Intern Med* on line, September 8, 2015.

29. Marmot, M. *The Health Gap: The Challenge of an Unequal World.* New York. *Bloomsbury*, 2015, 37, 263-264.

30. Woolhandler, S, Himmelstein, DU. When money is the mission: The high costs of investor-owned care. *New Engl J Med* 341: 444-446, 1999.

31. Churchill, LR. *Rationing health care in America: Perceptions and principles of justice.* Notre Dame, IN: University of Notre Dame, 1987.

32. Armour, S. Doctor-device deals need scrutiny, report says. *Wall Street Journal*, May 10, 2016: A3.

33. Williams, B. The ACA and the revolving door. *The Hill*. Available at htpp://thehill. com/blogs/congress-blog/healthcare/254556-the-ac...

34. Johnson, A. *Washington Post* ran 16 negative stories on Bernie Sanders in 16 hours. *Common Dreams*, March 8, 2016.

35. Hacker, JS, Pierson, P. *American Amnesia: How the War on Government Led Us to Forget What Made America Prosper.* New York. *Simon & Schuster,* 2016, pp.1-2.

36. Stiglitz, JE. Evaluating economic change. *Daedalus* 133/3, Summer, 2004.

37. Marmor, TR, Mashaw, JL, Pakutka, J. *Social Insurance: America's Neglected Heritage and Contested Future. Sage Copress.* Los Angeles, CA, 2014, p. 128.

38. Kuttner, R. Conservatives mugged by reality. *The American Prospect*, Jul/Aug 2014, p. 5.

CHAPTER 22

DIRECTIONS TOWARD
HEALTH CARE REFORM

Now that we have reflected on the major system changes in U.S. health care over the last 60 years, some positive, many negative, we come to the place where we need to chart directions to reform the system for the common good. From the preceding chapters, it is clear that the present system has been built to accommodate profiteering corporate stakeholders, not the needs of patients, and is unsustainable without major change.

So what are the main directions we should undertake to bring universal access to affordable health care in this country? In medicine and patient care, we like to start out with a problem list, in this case for the system itself. Therefore, this chapter has five goals: (1) to revisit the goals of medicine; (2) to consider non-partisan guiding principles for reform; (3) to list the major system problems we need to address; (4) to compare the three major alternatives of financing health care; and (5) to propose a problem-oriented action plan that medicine as a profession can adopt in leading toward patient-centered health care reform.

Goals of Medicine

A landmark study was undertaken by the Hastings Center in 1992 involving 14 countries ranging from Europe, Scandinavia, the United Kingdom, and the United States to Chile and China. It addressed where medicine has been, where it is going, and what its future priorities should be. Its 1996 comprehensive report, *The Goals of Medicine: Setting New Priorities,* is very relevant to health care reform 20 years later in this country. Table 22.1 lists the three goals that represent the core values of medicine and preserve the integrity of the medical profession in the face of political or social pressures. [1]

TABLE 22.1

Goals of Medicine

1. Prevention of Disease and Injury and Promotion and Maintenance of Health
2. Relief of Pain and Suffering Caused by Maladies
3. Care and Cure of Those with a Malady, and the Care of Those Who Cannot Be Cured

SOURCE: Project Report. *The Goals of Medicine: Setting New Priorities:* Special Supplement. Hastings Center Report, November-December, 1996:Executive Summary.

One of the difficult issues confronted by the participants in this study was how to prioritize curative vs. care goals of medicine. Their report framed the issue in these terms, still applicable today:

Although there is no inherent contradiction between care and cure, the bias toward the latter has often done harm to the former. The relentless and expensive wars against disease, particularly such lethal conditions as cancer, heart disease and stroke, have too often obscured the need for care and compassion in the face of mortality. Both the rate of technological innovation and its curative bias have created a medicine that is difficult to sustain, particularly in an equitable way. There is a limit to what can reasonably be paid for, what is politically feasible, and what market competition can sustain without great pain

*and inequity. The expansive, ambitious, open-ended pur-
suit of progress—the battles against illness that are never
quite won—that has been the mark of medicine over the
past fifty years may now have reached the boundaries of
perceived affordability in many countries.* [2]

Nonpartisan Conservative Guiding Principles
For Reform

The health care debate should be non-partisan. It is not a left-right issue, but has become a top-down issue in today's corporate dominated medical-industrial complex in a polarized political environment. Most conservatives in other advanced countries around the world have long accepted health care as a human right and built their health care systems on this basis. In his 1996 book, *Benchmarks for Fairness for Health Care Reform,* Donald Light, Ph.D, professor of comparative health care at the University of Medicine and Dentistry of New Jersey and researcher at the Edmond J. Safra Center for Ethics, noted that conservatives and business interests in every other industrialized country have endorsed these four conservative moral principles—*anti-free-riding, personal integrity, equal opportunity, and just sharing.* He proposed these 10 guidelines for conservatives to stay true to these principles:

1. *Everyone is covered, and everyone contributes in proportion to his or her income.*
2. *Decisions about all matters are open and publicly debated. Accountability for costs, quality and value of providers, suppliers, and administrators is public.*
3. *Contributions do not discriminate by type of illness or ability to pay.*
4. *Coverage does not discriminate by type of illness or ability to pay.*

5. *Coverage responds first to medical need and suffering.*

6. *Nonfinancial barriers by class, language, education and geography are to be minimized.*

7. *Providers are paid fairly and equitably, taking into account their local circumstances.*

8. *Clinical waste is minimized through public health, self-care, strong primary care, and identification of unnecessary procedures.*

9. *Financial waste is minimized through simplified administrative arrangements and strong bargaining for good value.*

10. *Choice is maximized in a common playing field where 90-95 percent of payments go toward necessary and efficient health services and only 5-10 percent to administration.* [3]

Problem List for U.S. Health Care

As we have seen in earlier chapters of this book, these are inter-related system problems in U.S. health care that need to be addressed:

1. Restricted access to care based on ability to pay.

2. More than 28 million uninsured Americans, with tens of millions underinsured.

3. Private health insurance with decreasing coverage and increasing cost.

4. Health insurance and health care increasingly unaffordable.

5. Loss of freedom of choice of physician, other providers, hospitals and other facilities.

6. An overly specialized physician workforce, with surpluses in many specialties and shortages in others.

7. Declining and inadequate primary care base.

8. Lack of a coherent plan for the future physician workforce.

9. Payment plans that encourage unnecessary and inappropriate care.

10. Market-based corporate profits that have replaced the service ethic of past years.

11. Uncontrolled escalation of health care costs and prices without cost containment in sight.

12. Lack of sufficient regulatory oversight to assure quality and effectiveness of health care services.

13. Increasing fragmentation and depersonalization of care.

14. Massive bureaucracy and administrative waste.

15. Increasing consolidation, market power, and lack of competition among providers and health care industries.

16. Increasing privatization of public programs, with tax dollars becoming corporate profits.

17. Poor comparisons for U.S. vs. other advanced countries in access, costs and quality of care.

18. Underfunding of public health and safety net programs.

19. A failed private health insurance industry that has been kept alive only by subsidies and permissive government policies.

Three Basic Financing Alternatives for Health Care

An informed, rational debate over health care in this country is long overdue. It should be based on our evidence-based experience with previous efforts to reform our system, not corporate money and lobbying of the vested interests in the status quo. Unfortunately, we did not have this debate in any substance during the 2016 election campaigns, with the exception of Bernie Sanders' important campaign issues.

We need fundamental financing reform, with three major alternatives:

1. Continuation of the Affordable Care Act (ACA) with marginal improvements.

Hillary Clinton ran on a platform committed to continuing the ACA, with these added modifications: adding the public option (which can't possibly succeed against the overwhelming market share of a subsidized insurance industry) [4], increasing subsidies, adding new tax credits for deductibles and co-payments not covered by insurance, lowering the age for Medicare eligibility to age 55, and empowering the government to negotiate drug prices. However, she ignored the fundamental flaws of the ACA, including the fact that, even when fully implemented, more than one-half of the previously uninsured population would remain uninsured. She seemed unable to acknowledge the declining value of insurance coverage, the flight of large insurers from the market, the loss of choice for patients, the continuing restricted access to care under the ACA, the increasing premium increases and profiteering by insurers, and the ACA's failure to contain costs or improve the quality of care. The three programs undertaken by the ACA to stabilize insurance premiums in revamped markets—reinsurance, risk corridors, and risk adjustment (the 3Rs)—have led to market instability, withdrawal of insurers from exchanges, and a flurry of lawsuits. [5]

The fourth 90-day open enrollment period that started on November 1, 2016 faced increased obstacles compared to earlier years—rising premiums, shrinking provider networks with less choice of physicians and hospitals, fewer options on the exchanges as major insurers left the market, and volatility of coverage. An additional problem for consumers was the refusal of some insurers, including Aetna and Cigna, to pay licensed agents and brokers to help people search for plans. [6] It appeared that no further reduction in the number of uninsured would take place. [7]

Clinton's frequently stated long-term goal of universal coverage was not credible, and is hypocritical in view of her 1994 statement of the inevitability of single-payer national health insurance by 2000 without health care reform. The ACA was never designed to get to universal coverage, which is impossible as long as the subsidized private health insurance industry remains in place.

2. Repeal and replacement of the ACA by a Republican "plan."

This has been a consistent goal of Republicans, starting soon after the passage of the ACA. That is easy to say, but the problem is that they still don't have a real plan for replacing it. The long-awaited "plan" released by House Republicans in June of 2016, a 37-page white paper called *A Better Way,* would rely on such long discredited features as consumer-directed health care, health savings accounts, selling insurance across state lines, and high risk pools. It would stop open-ended funding for Medicaid, institute block grants to states, and let states cut back coverage requirements under Medicaid. It would encourage businesses to band together to achieve more bargaining power in "Association Health Plans." It would also encourage further privatization of Medicare and would push traditional Medicare toward "premium support" vouchers with more control by private insurers. *A Better Way* would certainly increase the overall costs of health care, shift even more costs to patients, relieve corporate stakeholders of significant government oversight, while using tax monies without any projections of its cost to taxpayers. [8]

With less than three months to go before the election and with Trump plummeting in the polls, Republicans were gaming out a Plan B should Hillary Clinton win the presidency. They were working on a "grand bargain" by which states could have more flexibility through Section 1332 waivers to design market-based approaches to make insurance coverage more affordable (but of less value), while replacing the current ACA exchanges with their "innovative models." [9] The costs to taxpayers are unknown.

Republican governors in a number of states, including Arizona, Arkansas, Indiana, Iowa, Kentucky, Michigan, and Tennessee, have been submitting Medicaid waiver applications for federal approval by CMS that typically have premiums, co-pays, and one or another kind of health savings account. Some waiver applications include work requirements and incentives for specific health behaviors. Some have restricted coverage, such as for vision and dental care. Some terminate coverage for non-payment of premiums, with a required six-month lockout penalty, as in Kentucky. None of these proposals, however, are based on experience or evidence. [10] Instead, they fly in the face of studies that find that cost sharing in Medicaid programs is associated with missing or delaying needed care and worse outcomes, especially for people with chronic conditions. [11]

3. Single-payer national health insurance (NHI) or improved and expanded Medicare for All.

When and if NHI is enacted, all Americans will have universal access to affordable, comprehensive health care wherever they live and regardless of their income or health status. They will have free choice of physician and hospital. Their NHI cards will be good anywhere in the country (as is true in so many advanced countries around the world). Benefits will include physician and hospital care, outpatient care, dental services, vision services, rehabilitation, long-term care, home care, mental health care, and prescription drugs. Narrow networks will be gone. Medical bills will generally be eliminated, and patients will have no co-payments or other out-of-pocket costs at the point of service.

NHI will be funded through an equitable system of progressive taxation in which 95 percent of taxpayers will pay less than they do now for health insurance and care. A classic 2013 study by Gerald Friedman, professor of economics at the University of Massachusetts, projects the NHI will save $592 billion annually by cutting administrative waste of private insurers ($476 billion) and reducing pharmaceutical prices to European levels ($116 billion) through negotiated drug prices. These savings will allow all of the uninsured to be covered with upgraded benefits for all necessary care, and also fund $51 billion in transition costs, such as retraining displaced workers and phasing out investor-owned for-profit delivery systems over a 15-year period. Table 22.2 outlines the progressive financing plan for NHI, whereby, as examples, those with incomes of $50,000 would pay $1,500 a year in taxes, increasing to $6,000 for those with incomes of $100,000 and $12,000 for those with incomes of

TABLE 22.2

A Progressive Financing Plan For H.R. 676

This plan replaces regressive funding sources and improves and expands comprehensive benefits to all (in billions of dollars).

New progressive revenue sources

• Tobin tax of 0.5% on stock trades and 0.01% per year to maturity on transactions in bond, swaps, and trades.	442
• 6% surtax on household incomes over $225,000	279
• 6% tax on property income from capital gains, dividends, interest, or profits	310
• 6% payroll tax on top 60% with incomes over $53,000	346
• 3% payroll tax on bottom 40% with incomes under $53.000	27
Total new progressive sources	1,404
• Tax expenditure savings	260
• Federal Medicare, Medical, and other health spending, and 20% of current out-of-pocket spending (maintained from current system)	1.454
• Total Revenues	3,113
• Savings for deficit reduction	154

Source: Friedman, G. Funding H.R. 676 The Expanded and Improved Medicare For All Act. How We Can Afford a National Single Payer Health Plan. *Physicians for a National Health Plan.* Chicago, IL, July 31, 2013. Available at htpp://OHR%2067 6_Friedman_7.3.1.13.pdf

$200,000. [12] Compare this with the more than $25,000 per year that a typical family of four now pays for health insurance and care with an employer-based plan.

Private insurers will be banned from providing duplicative coverage to the public program, thus preventing them from lobbying for a two-tiered system that would underfund public coverage. NHI will be coupled with a private delivery system, and administered through a quasi-public entity. In no way is it socialized medicine, as its detractors like to say, with the government owning hospitals and other facilities and directly employing physicians and other health professionals.

Physicians in private practice will be paid based on a negotiated fee system, with increases for primary care physicians. Those working in non-profit hospitals, clinics, capitated group practices, HMOs, and integrated health systems will be salaried. Hospitals and other facilities will be paid through negotiated global budgets. An independent, non-partisan national scientific body will be established, free from political influence, to make evidence-based coverage decisions in the public interest. [13]

Table 22.3 compares the basic features of our three alternative financing systems. A modified ACA or the Republican "plan" will never resolve ongoing issues of access, affordability, and quality of health care. They have not, and cannot bring cost containment, will put a growing part of our population at an even worse position than they are today, and are unsustainable. [14]

TABLE 22.3

COMPARISON OF THREE REFORM ALTERNATIVES

	ACA	*GOP*	*NHI*
Access	Restricted	Restricted	Unrestricted
Choice	Restricted	Restricted	Unrestricted
Cost containment	No	No	Yes
Quality of care	Unimproved	Unimproved	Improved
Bureaucracy	Increased	Increased	Much reduced
Universal coverage	Never	Never	Immediately
Accountability	Limited	Limited	Yes
Sustainability	No	No	Yes

Table 22.4 shows how single-payer NHI is uniquely positioned to improve the quality of health care for all Americans, as conceptualized by Dr. Gordon Schiff, associate professor of internal medicine at Harvard Medical School. [15]

Despite marginal benefits of the ACA after almost seven years, a growing part of the population is left out, finds care unaffordable, and forgoes necessary care with poor outcomes that would be prevented under a system of universal coverage. We have to admit that the under-regulated health care marketplace, with its inefficient and wasteful multi-payer financing system, has failed. The market has proven itself unable and unwilling to meet the public interest. Only a larger role of government can accomplish that goal. Single-payer NHI is the only long-term solution to our problems, and is in keeping with traditional American values. (Table 22.5) [16]

Table 22.4

How Single-Payer NHI Will Improve Quality of Care

Access	• Everyone automatically eligible/ensured access; only plan for true universal insurance and access. • Able to control cost globally (w/ fences) so no reliance on access barriers to maintain affordability.
User-Friendly Simple	• A "no depends" system-no complicated rules, exchanges, variations by age, state, income, disease, employment/employer, marital status, etc. • Avoids eligibility determinations, means testing,confusion, enrollment complexities.
Single Standard	• By definition single system with fair rules for all • Generates database to identify disparities and track effectiveness of interventions
Continuity	• No switching for change in employment, divorce, new private insurance plan, restricted networks • Ensured reimbursement permitting provider financial stability.
Choice	• Avoids negative features and restricted networks, choice of provider and hospitals. • Uniform reimbursement and benefits package enables portability and ability to choose
Nursing	• Stable source of funding for hospitals via global budgets • Potentials for national standards, support for nursing education, less frustrations with arbitrary financially-driven anti-nurse cost cutting
Time	• All patients would be covered; ensuring provider is reimbursed for his/her time w/ each. • Greater potential for support of teamwork resulting from continuities of patients, staff, funding
Caring Commitment	• Elimination of greed, profit, corporate controls as the drivers health care system decision making • Restoring ability of professionals to advocate for patients and a better system, rather than current structured antagonisms
Clinical Information Systems	• Role and necessity of national standards, federal leadership in funding IT, demonstrated VA leadership, other countries lead • Design for clinical needs of patients, providers, not insurers, vendors (accountablity w/ unified system) • Ability to collect and aggregate data for quality oversight
Communication	• Better positioned to overcome trade secrets/secrecy inherent in private control • In avoiding financial barriers for patients to seek care, call, lower threshold/barriers for communication.
Continuous Improvement	• Stable public systems, "in business of health" for the long haul thus ROI on quality investment • Noteworthy successes of CQI in public sector (VA,Navy)
Accountability	• Public system by definition public & accountable, especially if democratic decision-making, organized advocacy efforts, vigilant media scrutiny, • Role that Medicare, Medicaid (and hence public insurance data) has played in outcomes evaluation and review of allocation decisions.
Prevention Oriented	• Unlike private plans where prevention does not pay due to frequent patient switches, greater incentives for prevention • Public system can be best integrated with public health at local and national levels

Table 22.5

Alternative Financing Systems and American Values

TRADITIONAL VALUE	Single-Payer	Multi-Payer
Efficiency	↑	↓
Choice	↑	↓
Affordability	↑	↓
Actuarial value	↑	↓
Fiscal responsibility	↑	↓
Equitable	↑	↓
Accountable	↑	↓
Integrity	↑	↓
Sustainable	↑	↓

Source: Geyman, JP. *Health Care Wars: How Market Ideology and Corporate Power Are Killing Americans*. Friday Harbor, WA. Copernicus Healthcare, 2012, p. 198.

A Problem-Oriented Action Plan for Medicine

In order to overcome the opposition of corporate interests in the medical-industrial complex and their lobbyists, a grassroots effort will be required to enact single-payer NHI. The medical profession can play an important leadership role in this direction. These are steps, from a physician's perspective, as put forward in my 2008 book, *The Corrosion of Medicine: Can the Profession Reclaim its Moral Legacy?*, that can usefully be taken by the profession in leading toward further necessary reforms of U.S. health care:

"• Reassert, through words and actions, that the raison d'etre of medicine is the health of patients and families, not the welfare of providers or their organizations.

- Assert our professionalism and independence in deciding which diagnostic, preventive, and therapeutic services to provide, based upon scientific evidence and cost-effectiveness, not on the marketing efforts by industry.
- Rein in flat-of-the-curve medicine (that with little proven value) in favor of a broader application of evidence-based medicine
- Embrace the chronic care model, with more temperate use of acute interventions when cure is not possible.
- Deal more directly with patients and their families about treatment options near the end of life, with greater sensitivity to patients' preferences.
- Be more skeptical of the claims of industry of effectiveness of new treatments and products, and require evidence of efficacy and cost-effectiveness before adopting new technologies.
- Expose and root out financial conflicts of interest of physicians and their organizations, including sanctions when necessary.
- Confront the profession's pervasive conflicts of interest with industry, and work towards more transparency and their elimination.
- Take more responsibility for the shortcomings of the system itself (and the profession's role in these problems).
- Become more knowledgeable about the problems of the health care system, and advocate for real health care reform.
- Take greater interest and become more involved in balancing the tension between population-based care and the care of individuals.
- Advocate for policies that achieve universal access to health care for the entire population, with reduction of disparities and inequities.
- Advocate for mental health parity (a 2006 review dispelled the old notion that this would lead to unaffordable over-utilization of health services). [17]

- Support policies to redress specialty and geographic maldistribution of physicians to best meet the needs of the public, with special emphasis on strengthening primary care at the base of the entire system and the care of underserved in urban and rural areas." [18]

Concluding Comment

Once Medicare for All is in place, physicians and other health care professionals will have more time to practice the way they were trained and committed. They will have more choices in how and where they will practice, and be relieved of some of today's pressures under their employers, especially large, consolidated hospital systems, to be more "productive" in bringing in more revenue. Small group practice will likely stage a comeback. Free from the burdens of dealing with the many private insurers and their changing bureaucratic requirements for such things as pre-authorizations of treatments and changing drug formularies, they will find their practices more satisfying with more time for direct patient care. Today's extensive administrative bureaucracy will be reduced and simplified. Most important, health care will become a right for all Americans, based on medical need, not ability to pay, and the quality of both individual and population care will improve immensely.

The recent observation by leaders of Physicians for a National Health Program, captures where we have been and need to go in U.S. health care:

> *Over the past century, myriad health care reforms— most well-intentioned—have been proposed and attempted. Yet, continued reliance on private insurers and profit-driven providers has doomed them to fail. It is time to chart a new course, to change the system itself. By doing so, we can realize, at last, the right to health care in America.* [19]

Endnotes:

1. Executive summary. Project Report. *The Goals of Medicine: Setting New Priorities.* Special supplement. *Hastings Center Report*, November-December 1996.

2. Ibid # 1, p. S4.

3. Light, DW. A conservative call for universal access to health care. *Penn J. Bioethics* 9 (4): 4-6, 2002.

4. Geyman, JP. Hillary's public option proposal: Could it work? *The Huffington Post*, June 3, 2016.

5. Adelberg, M, Bagley, N. Struggling to stabilize: 3Rs litigation and the future of the ACA exchanges. *Health Affairs Blog*, August 1, 2016.

6. Appleby, J. As insurers cut brokers' commissions, consumers may have one less tool for enrollment. *Kaiser Health News*, November 1, 2016.

7. Alonso-Zaldivar, R. CDC: Progress reducing uninsured rate threatens to stall. *Associated Press*, November 3, 2016.

8. Rovner, J. House Republicans unveil long-awaited plan to replace health law. *Kaiser Health News*, June 22, 2016.

9. Meyer, H. Could Trump loss spur ACA deal with Clinton? *Modern Healthcare*, August 6, 2016.

10. Grant, R. In Kentucky's new Medicaid plan evidence takes a back seat. *Health Affairs Blog*, August 25, 2016.

11. Issue Brief. The effect of premiums and cost sharing on access and outcomes for low-income children. *MACPAC,* July 2015.

12. Friedman, G. Funding H. R. 676: The Expanded and Improved Medicare for All Act. How We Can Afford a National Single-Payer Health Plan. *Physicians for a National Health Program.* Chicago, IL, July 31, 2013.

13. Gaffney, A, Woolhandler, S, Angell, M, Himmelstein, DU. Moving forward from the Affordable Care Act to a single-payer system. *Amer J Public Health* 106 (6): e1-2, June 2016.

14. Geyman, JP. *The Human Face of ObamaCare: Promises vs. Reality and What Comes Next.* Friday Harbor, WA. *Copernicus Healthcare*, 2016, p. 203.

15. Dr. Gordon Schiff. Personal communication, 2016.

16. Geyman, JP. *Health Care Wars: How Market Ideology and Corporate Power Are Killing Americans.* Friday Harbor, WA. *Copernicus Healthcare*, 2012, p. 198.

17. Barry, CL, Frank, RG, McGuire, TG. The costs of mental parity: still an impediment? *Health Affairs (Millwood)* 25 (3): 623-634, 2006.

18. Geyman, JP. *The Corrosion of Medicine: Can the Profession Reclaim its Moral Legacy?* Friday Harbor, WA. *Copernicus Healthcare*, 2008, 213-214.

19. Ibid # 9. Supplement to online version at http://www.ajphpublications.org/doi/pdf/10.2105/AJPH.2015.303157

CHAPTER 23
WHITHER THE FUTURE?

In my view, the provision of health care cannot continue to be dependent upon the whims and market projections of large private insurance companies whose only goal is to make as much profit as possible. That is why we need to join every other major country on earth and guarantee health care to all as a right, not a privilege. That is also why we need to pass a Medicare-for-all single-payer system.

—Senator Bernie Sanders, (I-VT), leader and proponent
of a new political revolution during his vigorous 2016
presidential campaign [1]

First they ignore you, then they laugh at you, then they fight with you, then you win.

— Mahatma Gandhi

Health care in America is at a crossroads. Where it goes from here is a huge and currently unanswerable political question. More than ever, it is a battle between private gain for the few against the common good of the many—the corporate, profit-driven stakeholders in our medical-industrial complex vs. the needs for essential health care of more than 320 million ordinary Americans.

The goals of this chapter are four-fold: (1) to describe how health care was dealt with during the 2016 election cycle; (2) to project the likely directions in health policy in the Trump administration and Republican-controlled Congress; (3) to summarize the continued chaos and impacts of "Trump Care" in our unraveling health care system; and (4) to consider prospects for future health care reform.

Health Care: A Major Issue during the 2016 election cycle

Going into the 2016 election campaigns, Democrats and progressives faced a steep hill to climb in order to gain the political power to be able to bring forward fundamental health care reform through single-payer national health insurance. They had to win the White House, as well as 30 seats in the House and 5 seats in the Senate in order to sweep Congress.

Bernie Sanders mounted a remarkable progressive campaign through and after the primaries on the Democratic side. Despite having campaign donations averaging just $27.00 against the well-bankrolled Clinton campaign, he brought in many millions of new voters, especially among millenials, with a level of energy far outpacing that of his rival.

After conceding the Democratic presidential nomination to Hillary Clinton, Bernie leveraged his political support to gain some progressive changes in the Democratic Party's Platform, including requiring Medicare to negotiate drug prices with Big PhRMA, expansion of community health centers, gaining Clinton's clear commitment to oppose the TPP, and support for a staged increase in the minimum wage. [2]

As a strong proponent of single-payer national health insurance (NHI), Medicare for All, here is how Bernie described the differences on the left and right on health care at the Democratic National Convention:

> *This campaign is about moving the United States to-ward universal health care and reducing the number of people who are uninsured or under-insured. Hillary Clin-ton wants to see that all Americans have the right to choose a public option in their health care exchange. She believes that anyone 55 years or older should be able to opt in to Medicare and she wants to see millions more Americans gain access to primary health care, dental care, mental health counseling and low-cost prescription drugs through a major expansion of community health centers.*
>
> *And what is Donald Trump's position on health care? No surprise there. Same old, same old Republican con-tempt for working families. He wants to abolish the Afford-able Care Act, throw 20 million people off of the health insurance they currently have and cut Medicaid for lower-income Americans.* [3]

Nowhere to be seen, however, was single-payer NHI, as Hillary continued her cautious and pragmatic ways while posturing reform as a "progressive" and vowing to "defend and expand" the ACA.

As the presidential race narrowed to two, Clinton vs. Trump, much was happening at the state level. The ACA itself had become a target of opportunity for Republicans as premiums for 2017 increased, networks further narrowed, big insurers exited major markets, and predictions of new enrollments on the exchanges fell far short of projections. Many Republicans gained ammunition for repeal of the ACA. By August 2015, the GOP-led House had already voted 56 times to repeal or undermine the ACA, but never developed a consensus plan to replace it. [4] Trump was campaigning on repeal of the ACA, saying that he would replace it with a "terrific plan."

Some Democrats, caught in tight re-election races, found their 2010 vote for the ACA a liability, especially in states that would decide which party will control the Senate in 2017, such as Arizona, Colorado, Indiana, North Carolina, Pennsylvania, and Wisconsin. Some Republicans jumped on the ACA's flaws, such as Senator John McCain of Arizona caught in a close re-election battle, running anti-Obamacare ads as state insurers raised premiums by as much as 88 percent and withdrew from many counties. [5] Meanwhile, the Koch brothers were pouring money into Colorado in an attempt to defeat ColoradoCare (Amendment 69), a single-payer proposal for universal health care on the November ballot with a broad base of support. [6]

Here is Jim Hightower's overall observation during mid-campaign about the single largest issue facing our country—the growing income and wealth inequality in our population, of which health care inequality is an important part:

> *The political cognoscenti have not understood the massive public rage over today's glaring inequality and mass downward mobility. This is a direct product of their wrenching the system with such power tools as "free" trade agreements, union busting, defunding public services, downsizing, offshoring, price gouging, Citizens United, privatization, the Wall Street bailout, student debt, tax dodging, criminalization of poverty, militarization of police . . . and so god-awful much more. . .*
>
> *No matter what happens to Sanders and Trump, the people who support them are not going away. The rebellion is on. Sanders and Trump are only the current messengers. The message itself is that We, the Grassroots People, now see that we're being sold out to giant corporations by our own leaders. Like the distant rumble of thunder, the boisterous uprising of outsiders in this year's election signals the approach of a historic storm. [7]*

Ralph Nader added this observation:

> *CBS president Leslie Moonves recently pulled no punches about the Trump phenomenon, saying it 'may not be good for America, but it's damn good for CBS'. . . . Trump is a symptom of a larger problem—profit-driven commercial television has put a stranglehold on our public discourse, highlighting controversy, carnage and entertainment fare over serious matters. The media industry reshaped our precious public commons into a fortress of exclusion that blocks dissenting, innovative and majoritarian viewpoints on matters that address society's basic needs. One thing is clear—something's gotta give.* [8]

Big Money played a major role in both the Democrat and Republican parties in determining the outcomes of the presidential and down-ballot campaigns. Financial ties with and conflicts of interest with the television and broadcast media have been well documented for the Clinton Foundation [9], while the workings of the Trump Foundation and Trump's financial dealings remain obscure and non-transparent, including refusal to release his tax returns.

The New Political Landscape and Health Care Reform
Implications of 2016 Election Results

The election results were a complete surprise to the establishments in both major parties, as well as for most public polls. Although Hillary Clinton won the popular vote by about 2.8 million votes, Donald Trump won more states than anyone predicted, emerging with an electoral college victory of 304 to 227. The Democrats gained two seats in the Senate, but the Republicans held their edge with 52 seats. In the House, the Republicans retained a big advantage, with 241 seats vs. 194 for the Democrats. At the state level, Republicans expanded their power to the strongest levels in decades, winning more than two-thirds of the nation's legislative chambers and 33 governors' offices. [10]

The Trump victory was a political earthquake felt all over the U.S. and overseas as well. Widespread protests took place in many cities across the country, with many people not trusting the president-elect or believing him unqualified. His authoritarian non-collaborative approach to the issues and racist bashing of minorities cast fear and anxiety across the land. Trump's emphasis on "law and order", with renewal of stop and frisk policies, exacerbated these fears. A number of far-right former leaders in Europe hailed his election as a forerunner of a growing right-wing wave stemming from shifts in the global economy, resurgent nationalism, racism and xenophobia, and eroding legitimacy of the mainstream media. [11]

These three perspectives shed light on the implications of the election results:

> *Trump's embrace of incivility (in addition to his embrace of racism and xenophobia) was a winning strategy, one that not only signaled the degree to which the politics of extremism has moved from the fringes to the center of American politics, but also one that turned politics into a spectacle that fed the rating machines [of the media]. . .*
>
> *What has been on full display in the presidential election of 2016 is the merging of the culture of cruelty, the logic of egregious self-interest, a deadly anti-intellectualism, a ravaging unbridled anger, a politics of disposability, and a toxic fear of others.* [12]

—Henry Giroux, Ph.D., McMaster University Professor for
Scholarship in the Public Interest and author of the 2015 book,
Dangerous Thinking in the Age of the New Authoritarianism

Exit polls reveal that the passionate support for Trump was inspired primarily by the belief that he represented change, while Clinton was perceived as the candidate who would perpetuate their distress. The "change" that Trump is likely to bring will be harmful or worse, but it is understandable that the consequences are not clear to isolated people in an atomized society lacking the kinds of associations (like unions) that can educate and organize. That is a crucial difference between today's despair and the generally hopeful attitudes of many working people under much greater economic duress during the Great Depression of the 1930s. [13]

—Noam Chomsky, Ph.D., professor emeritus of linguistics at
the Massachusetts Institute of Technology, and co-author of
Profits Over People: Neoliberalism and Global Order

It is hard to contemplate the new administration without experiencing alarm bordering on despair: Alarm about the risks of war, the fate of constitutional democracy, the devastation of a century of social progress. Trump's populism was a total fraud. Every single Trump appointment has come from the pool of far-right conservatives, crackpots, and billionaire kleptocrats. More alarming still is the man himself—his vanity, impulsivity, and willful ignorance, combined with an intuitive genius as a demagogue. A petulant fifth-grader will now control the awesome power of the U. S. government. [14]

—Robert Kuttner, Ph.D., co-editor of *The American
Prospect* and author of *Everything for Sale:
The Virtues and Limits of Markets*

This election cycle has left us with a more polarized country than ever. Trump's campaign was enabled by many Republicans as well as the media that gave free airtime to his wild non-factual assertions as "the latest news" with little accountability for the truth. He brought an ugly combination of racism, xenophobia, bigotry, misogyny, fear mongering, and white nationalism to the forefront. Living in Trump Tower and disconnected from the working class, Trump postured himself as an outsider and leader of a new populist movement. Surprisingly, he gained widespread support from an angry, alienated electorate (some of whom even crossed party lines) that bought into his simplistic solutions to national problems. Especially noteworthy was the wide split in the rural-urban vote, with red covering almost all of rural America. As Robert Reich points out, the Democratic party itself was also complicit in the Trump victory, having largely abandoned the working class over the last two decades and becoming beholden to corporate and Wall Street money. [15]

ACA Controversy and Public Concerns

The ACA was one of the key issues debated throughout a highly polarized, mostly negative campaign, with all Republican candidates arguing for its repeal. The sharp spikes in insurance premiums for 2017 became a hot issue towards the end of the campaign. As expected, corporate money played a big role in the results, including in state initiatives, where we saw Proposition 61 in California (intended to control drug prices by requiring discounts as the VA does)[16] and Colorado's Amendment 69, ColoradoCare (a single-payer initiative), soundly defeated.

A Reuters poll taken nine days after the election found health care to be the top issue that Americans wanted Trump to address in the first 100 days of his administration, even above jobs. [17] Two weeks later, however, a Kaiser Health Tracking Poll found widespread disagreement among responders about what to do about the ACA, with 30 percent favoring its expansion, 26 percent wanting its repeal, 19 percent continuing it as is, and 17 percent wanting to scale it back. [18] According to the Quinnipiac University National Poll in early January, only 42 percent of responders were optimistic about the next four years. [19] Meanwhile, a *Wall Street Journal/NBC* poll in mid-January found Trump's favorable ratings fall to a low of 38 percent, the lowest for a president-elect in polling history and far below president-elect Obama's 67 percent during his transition. [20] A Pew Research Center poll at the same time showed that 60 percent of Americans say the government should be responsible for ensuring health care coverage for all Americans, up from 51 percent in 2016. [21] One week after Trump's inauguration, an Associated Press-NORC Center for Public Affairs Research found that 56 percent of U. S. adults were "extremely" or "very" concerned about losing their health insurance if the ACA is repealed, including 45 percent of Republicans as "somewhat" concerned. [22]

The election of Vice-President Pence and other announcements of key Cabinet appointments do not bode well for the future of U.S. health care. As Governor of Indiana, Mike Pence expanded Medicaid under Indiana's HIP 2.0 waiver. It imposed payments on enrollees, even those below the poverty level, as "skin in the game," established Personal Wellness and Responsibility (POWER) accounts, and required individuals who failed to keep up their contributions to lose coverage. [23] Seema Verma, president and CEO of a health policy consulting company and Trump's pick to head the Centers for Medicare and Medicaid (CMS) with its almost $1 trillion annual budget, helped to implement HIP 2.0 in Indiana as well as similar programs in other states. As the new head of Indiana's Medicaid program, she shifted all Medicaid recipients at once to private managed care; nine months later, widespread complaints were coming in from hospitals, nursing homes, and clinics about losses of hundreds of thousands of dollars in expected payments. [24] According to the *Indianapolis Star*, she received millions of dollars through the Indiana state government as well as more than $500 million from Hewlett-Packard, a Medicaid vendor, in state contracts, considered by ethics experts as conflicts of interest. [25]

Then Trump selected Dr. Tom Price, orthopedic surgeon and Rep-GA, current chairman of the House Budget Committee, and co-founder of the conservative Congressional Tea Party caucus, as the incoming head of the Department of Health and Human Services. He authored the *Empowering Patients First Act* as a replacement for the ACA, which would do away with mandated coverage, promote a free-market approach, fully repeal Medicaid expansion, eliminate the ACA's requirement for coverage of essential services, add tax credits, and give insurers wide latitude to charge older enrollees as much as they want. [26] Although he had an obvious conflict of interest revealed during his confirmation hearings over purchase of biomedical stocks at a discounted price as a member of Congress passing supportive legislation for such companies [27], he was confirmed by a party line vote for his new post. Price's appointment also foretells the GOP's plans to privatize both Medicare and Medicaid, which now serve about 57 million elderly and disabled Americans and 77 million low-income people. [28]

The GOP's Dilemma on Health Care

Now that it has control of the White House and both chambers of Congress, the GOP has a conundrum, much like the dog that caught the bus. Republicans are telling us that they will bring us "universal access to health care and coverage," stating that their goal is "to make sure that everybody can buy coverage or find coverage if they choose to." (my emphasis). [29] What deception that is!

On Inauguration Day, President Trump issued an Executive Order urging federal officials "to take all actions consistent with the law to minimize the unwarranted economic and regulatory burdens" of the ACA. [30] He also called for "the States to be given more flexibility and control to create a more free and open health market." No details were provided as Congress was called upon to expeditiously repeal and replace the ACA. [31]

But the GOP has a big problem—it has several competing plans for the ACA's replacement without any consensus among their proponents as to timing of its repeal. Alternative replacement plans include Paul Ryan's *Better Way,* Tom Price's *Empowering Patients First Act*, and the *Patient Freedom Act of 2017*, introduced by Senators Susan Collins (R-ME) and Bill Cassidy (R-LA). At their three-day policy retreat in late January titled *Keeping Our Promise on Health Care*, Republicans were far from any agreement on how to go forward and very concerned about not having a replacement plan ready when the ACA was repealed.

Rather than expecting a single replacement for the ACA, it appears that we will see a combination of changes through a budget reconciliation bill requiring just 51 votes in the Senate, regulatory action and executive orders by the Trump administration, and individual bills addressing smaller aspects of the health system. [32] One such bill has just been introduced in the House that is intended to preserve the ACA's protections requiring insurers not to deny coverage on the basis of pre-existing conditions. [33] Instead of early action on the ACA, Paul Ryan's goal is to pass repeal legislation by August 2017, despite pressure from the White House. [34] As Republican legislators confronted the complexity of their repeal and replace strategy, some were shifting toward a "repair" approach to the ACA's problems. [35] As Tom MacArthur (R-NJ) said after their three-day retreat:

> *We'd better be sure that we're prepared to live with the market we've created . . . That's going to be called 'Trumpcare', and Republicans will own that lock, stock and barrel, and we'll be judged in the election less than two years away.* [36]

As Republicans confronted the difficulties and political hazards of repealing the ACA, their confusion and lack of consensus over next steps increased as they delayed their timetables. Even President Trump had to admit that his high priority to fix health care "was becoming a drawn-out Washington process that could stretch for months or even years."

Should they repeal the ACA altogether, Republicans will have to answer politically for adding 20 million Americans to the rolls of the uninsured (including about 15 million through expanded Medicaid) as well as ending such popular provisions as requirements that insurers offer coverage without regard to pre-existing conditions and allowing children up to age 26 on their parents' policies.[37] They would likely be opposed by governors in states that expanded Medicaid under the ACA, who would feel the direct anger of former beneficiaries. Democratic governors have warned Congress that repeal of the ACA will cost them almost $69 billion in costs for uncompensated care over the next ten years. [38] Republicans would also own widespread public anger when some of their pet proposals in their "plan" encounter public resistance. Just three weeks into the new Trump administration, a Public Policy Poll found widespread resistance to the ACA's repeal, with 47 percent supporting the ACA and only 39 percent opposed, as well as an approval rating for Trump of just 43 percent compared to 53 percent disapproving. [39] Widespread protests to the GOP's approach to health care were already occurring across the country.

A replacement plan will be technically difficult and potentially politically explosive, and will require at least 60 votes in the Senate to pass, including some Democratic support. During an extended period before the GOP can come up with a replacement plan, we can anticipate increasingly widespread anxiety and uncertainty among patients, their families, and insurers. We can also expect growing instability of the insurance market as insurers leave the market in droves. [40]

With Tom Price heading up the Department of Health and Human Services, he has wide latitude to implement some of the GOP's agenda for health care by rule changing, thereby not requiring action by Congress. As examples, he could stop enforcing the individual mandate, give insurers more flexibility to determine what health benefits they will or won't pay for, and more strictly monitor new ACA enrollees. Such moves would likely make it harder for people to get coverage for maternity and mental health care, while undoing the ACA's standard requiring contraceptive coverage as a preventive health benefit. [41]

Another important part of the fallout of Republicans taking on health care "reform" will be strong pushback from the insurance and hospital industries that have benefitted so much from expanded markets under the ACA. Trump's election ignites great uncertainty for health insurers across all of their markets—individual, employer-based, ACA exchanges, Medicare and Medicaid. Their stocks took an immediate hit right after the election. The ACA has been a Faustian bargain whereby the Obama administration needed a cooperative insurance industry, and that interdependence still stands as the Republicans consider doing away with it, thereby stranding millions of Americans without insurance. In the negotiations to come, the industry still has a big stick by saying it will just exit markets unless the government keeps paying even more for its continued involvement. It keeps threatening the specter of its own "death spiral" unless it receives an ongoing bailout by the government.

One example of the insurance industry's concern were Medicaid-centric insurers, such as Centene, Molina Healthcare, and WellCare Health Plans, which worried that their growth in Medicaid enrollees would come to a halt. [42] Without the ACA, hospitals will have to confront the loss of millions of previously insured patients at a time of rising costs and an aging population. [43] The American Hospital Association and the Federation of American Hospitals have warned that repeal of the ACA will cost hospitals $165 billion by the middle of the next decade and lead to "an unprecedented public health crisis." [44]

In effect, whatever health care "reforms" the Republicans put in place in coming months, a larger and growing part of the population will find necessary health care inaccessible and/or unaffordable, stoking increasing public outrage. At the same time, it will be harder for the Republican-led administration to meet the needs of the private health insurance industry, which has thrived under the ACA and which is not sustainable without increasing government support.

If the GOP proceeds to try to privatize Medicare further, as both Paul Ryan and Tom Price have called for, they will encounter enormous backlash from seniors and Democrats. Some Republican leaders are already seeing that as a third rail to be avoided as Democrats welcome it as a wedge issue for the 2018 midterm elections.

In this period of political uncertainty, Michael Lind, co-founder of the New America Foundation, sees the major alternative for financing health care this way:

> *The U.S. health insurance system is likely to move either toward efficient social insurance or toward inefficient and costly voucherization of the social insurance elements*

like Medicare and Medicaid, combined with rationing of health care of a kind unknown in other advanced industrialized democracies. For reasons of solvency and fairness alike, health insurance needs to be absorbed into an expanded, comprehensive American social insurance system.[45]

Prognosis: Increasing Chaos of "Trump Care" as our Health Care System Unravels Further

According to the National Center for Health Statistics, even as it struggled along, the ACA wasn't working for more than 28 million uninsured and tens of millions underinsured individuals. After almost seven years, it reduced the number of uninsured by less than one-half. Most adults under age 65 were still insured by their employers, but that coverage was becoming more meager each year with higher and higher cost sharing. Less than 5 percent of the insured have received coverage through the ACA's exchanges, far short of all earlier projections. For those under age 65, high-deductible health plans increased from 25 percent in 2010 to 40 percent in 2016, putting added financial pressure on patients trying to afford needed care. [46] Since 2011, average deductibles for single coverage in employer health plans soared by 63 percent. [47]

Based on existing trends and aggravated by likely incremental "reforms" taken by the new administration and Congress, the power of the unchecked private health insurance industry will continue as it battles hospitals, physician groups, and other players in an ongoing private marketplace designed for profits, not service to patients. Robert Reich sees our post-election future this way:

Health insurers spend lots of time, effort, and money trying to attract people who have high odds of staying healthy (the young and fit) while doing whatever they can

327

to fend off those who have high odds of getting sick (the older, infirm, and unfit). As a result we end up with the most bizarre health-insurance system imaginable: One ever more carefully designed to avoid sick people. . . . In reality, they're becoming very big to get more bargaining leverage over everyone they do business with—hospitals, doctors, employers, the government, and consumers. That way they make even bigger profits. [48]

Whether the ACA is repealed, partly dismantled, "repaired," or replaced with Republican proposals, what we can count on is worse access to affordable health care, ongoing inequities and disparities, and increasing waste and bureaucracy as corporate stakeholders in our market-based system further increase their profits on the backs of the sick and taxpayers. Given the opportunity, insurers will go back to their old ways, including charging women higher insurance premiums than men, overcharging seniors, issuing worthless bare-bones policies, and exiting unprofitable markets. [49]

We can also expect to see large increases in the numbers of un-insured and underinsured Americans, reduced utilization and funding of the nation's hospitals, further erosion of safety net programs, new threats to Medicare and Medicaid, harmful impacts on women's health care if Planned Parenthood is defunded, and worsening health outcomes for both individuals and our population. Repeal of the ACA would result in at least 20 million Americans losing their health insurance, with an estimated 43,000 deaths annually. [50] As health policy experts Drs. Himmelstein and Woolhander predict, the likeliest replacement of the ACA will be "a meaner (and rebranded) facsimile of the ACA that retains its main structural element—us-ing tax dollars to subsidize private insurance—while imposing new burdens on the poor and sick." [51] Figure 23.1 illustrates what we can expect with "Trump Care."

FIGURE 23.1

Trump's Health Care "Plan"

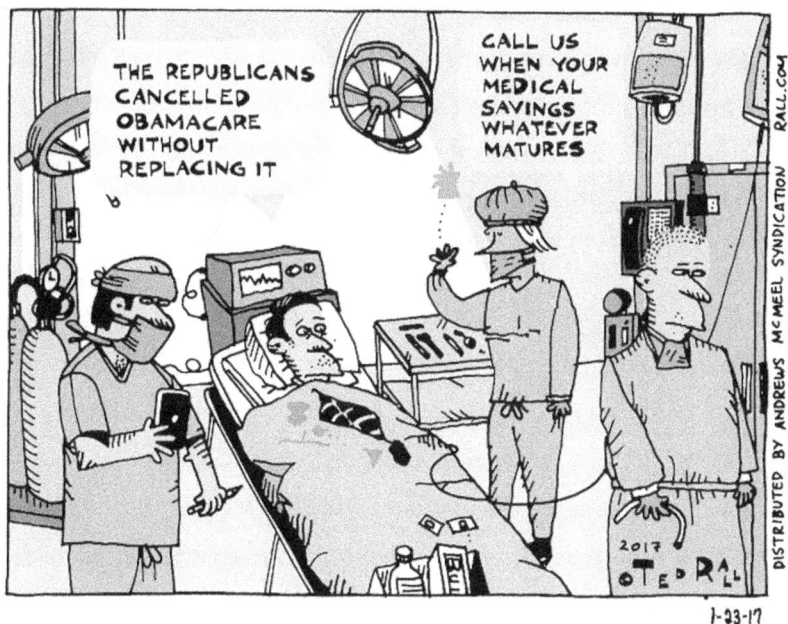

Source: Reprinted with permission of the artist, Ted Rall

These continuing and accelerating trends all lead to unsustainability sooner than later. We will come to the point where we must replace the predatory, multi-payer financing system with a not-for-profit public financing system—single-payer NHI—coupled with a more accountable private delivery system. Dr. Jack Geiger, who developed the community health center movement and dedicated his medical career to social justice, at 90 and blind, recently stated:

You don't need eyesight to hold on to a vision. [52]

329

The Road Ahead: Real Reform is Inevitable, Just a Matter of Time

Essential Changes Needed

1. **We need news media dedicated to speaking truth to power and committed to the common good.** *Truthout* is a classic example of a publication that does just that. Mike Ludwig, one of its staff reporters, recently observed:

   > *The functional divide between the mainstream media and our publication has never been clearer. The corporate media profited from the rise of an autocrat, and in turn provided Trump with billions in free advertising. Now that Trump has seized power, the corporate media is already working to normalize him and his cohorts, and will be all too happy to frame his antics as good television. As we enter this period of uncertainty, we can no longer afford to pretend that major news outlets have any capacity to serve the truth, or the interests of those marginalized by people like Trump. Our work will be more necessary than ever, and may be more perilous than ever.* [53]

2. **Democrats have to learn from the election and change.** They have supported the social institutions of neoliberalism for decades, welcomed corporate money in their campaigns, and largely abandoned the working class, as shown by the revolt in 2016 of voters in the Rust Belt states. [54]

3. **Single-payer health care reform organizations need to participate actively in broader coalitions that span many progressive issues in order to gain political power and influence.** These efforts should be focused on the harms being inflicted on a growing part of our population by corporate greed of the medical-industrial complex and related corporate allies.

In their 2016 book, *Nation on the Take: How Big Money Corrupts Our Democracy and What We Can Do About It*, Wendell Potter, senior analyst at the Center for Public Integrity, and Nick Penniman, director of the Huffington Post Investigative Fund, bring us this historical perspective:

> *America's last Gilded Age gave rise to rebellious fires, the flames of which eventually spread to Teddy, a well-to-do Republican and progressive who was the single greatest champion of campaign finance reform this country has ever seen. He didn't believe in reform as an end in itself. He saw it as a means to reclaim the right to self-government, and the right for every person to have an equal opportunity to get ahead in life—what he termed a "square deal."* [55]

Thomas Jefferson would have agreed. In a letter to James Madison in 1787, he said:

> *I hold it that a little rebellion now and then is a good thing, and as necessary in the political world as storms in the physical.* [56]

Both the Sanders and Trump campaigns revealed a spreading wave of public anger, albeit from different populist perspectives, over the present system, where big money and political power undermine our democracy. Hedrick Smith, Pulitzer Prize-winning former *New York Times* reporter, points to two trigger points to populist backlash: the Supreme Court's Citizens United decision and the GOP's "Roadmap" strategy that enabled the Republican Party to take control of enough state governments in 2010 to gerrymander its way to a 33-seat majority in the House of Representatives in 2012, even though Democratic candidates for the House received 1.5 million more votes. [57]

Some important questions going forward

- Could President Donald Trump, priding himself on unpredictability, supposedly less beholden to corporate money, and with a business view of health care, surprise Americans in coming around to single-payer national health insurance? His opening pledge is to be the president for all Americans. Among his many contradictory views expressed on health care in past years, he has noted the advantages of single-payer universal coverage in other countries such as Canada and Scotland. If he did so today, he could garner the support of much of the electorate on both sides of the aisle and give his divided party an issue with strong popular support for generations to come.

- Is it possible that more Republicans will come around to NHI, given the failures of the ACA and the lack of a positive alternative plan supported by the public? A Gallup poll in May 2016 found that 41 percent of Republicans and leaners favored replacing the ACA with Medicare for All. [58]

- Will more Republicans in Congress and conservative business leaders recognize the four conservative moral principles described in the last chapter that support NHI and are supported by most advanced nations around the world?

- Will more large employers come to welcome giving up the burden of ESI and gaining a healthier workforce which costs them less?

- Will small business do likewise? A majority of small business owners in California, for the first time in years of surveys, supported Medicare for All in 2016. [59]

- Will a powerful national women's movement succeed in pushing back GOP attempts to restrict their choices of contraception and access to legal abortion?

Another important question is how much the new GOP health care plan will cost. Suffice it to say, nobody knows, except that we can be sure that it will cost patients, families and taxpayers far more than expected. Disingenuously, the House Republicans passed a rule less than two weeks before Trump's inauguration banning the Congressional Budget Office (CBO) from reporting a cost analysis of the ACA's repeal and its impact on the deficit. That will allow the GOP to skirt a law requiring their 2017 ACA repeal legislation to expire in 10 years without an independent CBO cost analysis. [60]

Based on an earlier cost analysis of the GOP's Restoring Americans' Healthcare Freedom Reconciliation Act of 2015 (considered a likely prototype of a partial repeal of the ACA), the Congressional Budget Office and Joint Committee on Taxation have recently estimated that elimination of the ACA's Medicaid expansion and marketplace subsidies would double premiums and increase the number of uninsured by 32 million by 2026. They also projected that insurers would likely stop offering coverage in the individual market, with about half of the population living in areas without any insurer in the non-group market in the first year after repeal of marketplace subsidies. [61] A recent independent study by the Commonwealth Fund and George Washington University's Milken School of Public Health concludes that repeal of both federal premium tax credits and Medicaid expansion without a viable alternative will lead to a $140 billion cut in federal funding by 2019, which would "trigger losses in employment, economic activity, and state and local revenues"; that study estimates that there will be, between 2019 and 2023, a cumulative $1.5 trillion loss in gross state products and a $2.6 trillion reduction in business output. [62]

Republicans will own whatever they do in 2017 and 2018. They will almost certainly face a powerful political backlash as more Americans can't afford coverage and care. That can be a big political opportunity for a chastened and re-energized Democratic party to carry the day in the 2018 midterms, regain control of Congress, and develop momentum for a landslide return to power in the 2020 election cycle through the leadership of progressive candidates.

Some promising trends

A number of new developments in the post-election political environment and the early days of the Trump administration offer hope for progressive change in health care. Bernie Sanders has announced the formation of "Our Revolution" to support progressive candidates up and down the ticket. Sanders' organizers have already launched a national, volunteer-led Brand New Congress (BNC), with plans to run at least 400 progressive candidates for Congress in 2018, financed by small, crowd-sourced donations. [63] Based on their experience in watching the rise of the Tea Party, former congressional staffers have pulled together an important document, *Indivisible: A Practical Guide for Resisting the Trump Agenda*, to encourage grassroots resistance across the country based on values of inclusion, tolerance, and fairness. [64] At the state level, 17 states and more than 680 local governments have appealed to Congress for a constitutional amendment to overturn Citizens United. [65]

Jim Hightower sees our future political battles this way:

> *By continuing to organize and mobilize across the country around populist issues and local campaigns, the uprising sparked by Sanders is the future of American politics. The Working Families Party, the Greens, the majority of Democrats (including Hillary backers), and the no-party people are in open rebellion against the moneyed plutocracy, and change is coming. To advance it, thousands of us Berniecrats have launched Our Revolution, an independent, state-based political network that flows from, and is building on, the progress and grassroots structures*

of Sanders' seminal run. It's already organizing for next year's local elections and looking toward the 2018 congressional races, the 2020 presidential contest—and beyond. Link up at www.ourrevolution.org. [66]

The prognosis for NHI could be much improved in the next few years as the ACA (if still alive) and public dissatisfaction with health care reaches a widespread backlash across party lines and as the forces for progressive change gain further strength. The 2018 midterm elections could further increase the numbers of progressive legislators in Congress, and potential presidential candidates such as Elizabeth Warren could provide new impetus toward needed reform in the 2020 election cycle.

In their 2016 book, *American Amnesia: How the War on Government Led Us to Forget What Made America Prosper*, political scientists Jacob Hacker and Paul Pierson give us this optimistic view of where we now are:

> *[If we take on] the modern robber barons of health care, finance, energy, and other sectors, we can generate even bigger benefits—from slower growth of health spending to lower pollution, from longer lives to stronger financial security, from increased educational opportunity to decreased economic hardship. In short, there is money on the table just waiting to be picked up. At a time when so many argue that we live in an age of inherent limits, we have something truly exciting to aim for: We can make our already prosperous society much more prosperous. And in doing so, we can also get our troubled democracy back on track. Right now American politics is dominated by narrow interests and driven by zero-sum conflicts.* [67]

As our health care system continues to implode, medicine as a profession has new opportunities to lead toward health care reform and reclaim its leadership role and moral legacy from earlier years. Physicians and their organizations have more potential power to guide system reform than they may think. Some organizations have already played a major role, such as Physicians for a National Health Program (PNHP), with more than 22,000 physicians in all specialties, which published its most recent proposal in 2016 for single-payer NHI. [68] Other proactive medical organizations working toward universal access to health care include leaders of the American College of Physicians, the American Psychiatric Association, and the American Society of Clinical Oncology. Even the ever-reactionary American Medical Association, long resistant to universal health care, could come around to NHI when they see the wreckage that the GOP has wrought over health care. In early January of 2017, Dr. Howard Bauchner, the Editor in Chief of its journal, JAMA, has recently stated:

> *All physicians, including those who are members of Congress, other health care professionals, and professional societies (should) speak with a single voice and say that health care is a basic right for every person, and not a privilege to be available and affordable only for a majority.* [69]

Other health professionals have already taken strong leadership roles toward reform, especially prominent members of the American Nurses Association, the American Public Health Association, and National Nurses United. All health professionals need to recognize and use their political power—there can be no patient care without them and their health care teams. The system comes to a halt without them— administrators cannot care for patients!

Concluding Comment

Today's health care system, serving its corporate masters more than patients, is unfair, ineffective, inhumane for those left out, and financially unsustainable. Fundamental financing reform is inevitable, and is required sooner than later. We can take heart from these words by the late Dr. Quentin Young, tenacious advocate for social justice in health care and author of *Everybody In Nobody Out: Memoirs of a Rebel Without a Pause*:

> *From my adolescent years to the present, I've never wavered in my belief in humanity's ability—and our collective responsibility—to bring about a more just and equitable social order. I've always believed in humanity's potential to create a more caring society. . . I retain a terrible reputation for excessive optimism. The glories of humankind's ingenuity and inventiveness have not yet been exhausted. The future can be bright, but only if we work to make it so.* [70]

Endnotes:

1. Sanders, B. Sanders' statement on Aetna's decision to withdraw from health insurance exchanges. August 16, 2016.
2. Hightower, J. What's the next Bernie Sanders revolution? *The Progressive Populist*, August 15, 2016, p. 3.
3. Boggioni, T. Here is the full text of Bernie Sanders' speech at the 2016 Democratic National Convention, *Raw Story*, July 25, 2016.
4. Fahrenthold, DA, Johnson, J. Republicans' Obamacare 'repeal and replace' dilemma joins presidential contest. *The Washington Post*, August 18, 2015.
5. Pradhan, R. Demko, P. Obamacare sticker shock hits key Senate races. *Politico*, August 26, 2016.
6. Corcoran, M. Koch brothers attempt to kill single-payer health care in Colorado. *Truthout*, March 24, 2016.

7. Hightower, J. The uprising of the outsiders. *The Hightower Lowdown*, July/August 2016.

8. Nader, R. The need for progressive voices. *Common Dreams*, May 6, 2016.

9. Corcoran, M. The Clinton Foundation and the media: A deep-seated conflict of interest. *Truthout*, September 1, 2016.

10. *Associated Press*, Republicans expand control of governorships, legislatures. New York Times, November 9, 2016.

11. Harvey, R. Rising European fascists welcome Trump victory. *Truthout*, November 12, 2016.

12. Giroux, HA. The authoritarian politics of resentment in Trump's America. *Truthout*, November 13, 2016.

13. Chomsky, N. as quoted by Polychroniou , CJ. Trump in the White House: An Interview with Noam Chomsky. *Truthout*, November 14, 2016, p. 6.

14. Kuttner, R. The audacity of hope. *The American Prospect*, Winter 2017, pp. 5-7.

15. Reich, R. Trump's three enablers: The GOP, the Media, and . . . the Establishment Democrats. *Common Dreams*, November 8, 2016.

16. Johnson, CY. Drug companies just scored a big victory. *The Washington Post,* November 9, 2016.

17. Kahn, C. Americans want Trump to focus on healthcare first: Poll. *Reuters*, November 17, 2016.

18. Kirzinger, A, Sugarman, E, Brodie, M. Kaiser Health Tracking Poll. *Kaiser Family Foundation*, November 2016.

19. Tamias blog. Donald Trump's approval rating nose-dive. *Daily Kos*, January 11, 2017.

20. Hook, J. Trump's popularity slips. *Wall Street Journal*, January 18, 2017: A6.

21. Bialik, K. More Americans say government should ensure health care coverage. Pew Research Center, January 13, 2017.

22. Alonzo-Zalvidar, R, Swanson, E. AP-NORC poll: Broad worries about potential health care loss. *U. S. News,* January 27, 2017.

23. Galewitz, P. Pence expanded health coverage as Governor, now threatens to take it away. *Kaiser Health News*, November 28, 2016.

24. Harper, J. Trump's pick to run Medicare and Medicaid has red state policy chops. *Kaiser Health News*, November 29, 2016.

25. *IndyStar*. Powerful state healthcare consultant serves two bosses. August 25, 2014.

26. Kliff, S. By picking Tom Price to lead HHS, Trump shows he's absolutely serious about dismantling Obamacare. *Vox*, November 28, 2016.

27. Blumenthal, P. Contrary to sworn testimony, company confirms Trump's HHS pick got special stock deal. *The Huffington Post*, January 30, 2017.

28. Rovner, R. Price's appointment boosts GOP plans to overhaul Medicare and Medicaid. *Kaiser Health News*, November 29, 2016.

29. Pear, R, Kaplan, T. Republicans' deceptive concept of 'universal access.' *New York Times*, December 15, 2016.

30. Rovner, J. Trump's first order has strong words on health. Actual impact may be weak. *Kaiser Health News*, January 24, 2017.

31 Brunetti, JK. Trump's Executive Order on the ACA and future compliance obligations. *ACA Times*, January 23, 2017.

32. Rovner, J. At party retreat, GOP still searching for health law consensus. *Kaiser Health News*, January 26, 2017.

33. Sullivan, P. GOP chairman to introduce pre-existing conditions bill. *The Hill,* January 26, 2017.

34. House, B. Republicans are making little progress on their Obamacare repeal strategy. *Bloomberg.com*, January 27, 2017.

35. Sullivan, P. GOP talk shifts from replacing ObamaCare to repairing it. *The Hill*, February 1, 2017.

36. Associated Press. Republican lawmakers worry if 'Trumpcare' doesn't deliver. *The Washington Post*, January 28, 2017.

37. Shear, MD, Pear, R. From 'repeal' to 'repair': Campaign talk on health law meets reality. *New York Times*, February 6, 2017.

38. Scott, D. Can Trump kill Obamacare? He'll have to answer these questions first. *STAT*, November 9, 2016.

39. Americans now evenly divided on impeaching Trump. *Public Policy Polling*, February 10, 2017.

40. *Associated Press.* Democratic governors warn Congress on health care repeal. December 21, 2016.

41. Cancryn, A, Demko, P. Obamacare repeal plan stokes fears of market collapse. *Politico*, November 21, 2016.

42. Herman, B. Trump, GOP sweep may disrupt every corner of health insurance industry. *Modern Healthcare*, November 9, 2016.

43. Hancock, J, Luthra, S. Obamacare 'replacement' might look familiar. *Kaiser Health News*, November 9, 2016.

44. *Associated Press.* Democratic governors warn Congress on health care repeal. December 21, 2016.

45. Lind, M. The next social contract. *New America Foundation*, 2013.

46. Cohen, RA, Martinez, ME, Zammitti, EP. Health insurance coverage: Early release of estimates from the first quarter of the *2016 National Health Interview Survey*, January-March 2016, September 2016. Washington, D.C. *National Center for Health Statistics*.

47. Hancock, J, Luthra, S. Studies: Employer costs slow as consumers use less care, deductibles soar. *Kaiser Health News*, September 14, 2016.

48. Reich, R. Why a single-payer health care system is inevitable. *The Huffington Post*, August 28, 2016.

49. Potter, W. Regardless of who we vote for, health insurers will win. *Wendell Potter blog*, November 4, 2016.

50. Himmelstein, DU, Woolhandler, S. Repealing the Affordable Care Act will kill more than 43,000 people annually. *The Washington Post*, January 23, 2017.

51. Woolhandler, S, Himmelstein, DU. Health reform in the Trump era: A big step back, but possibilities for bigger steps forward. *Physicians for a National Health Program*. Chicago, IL, November 16, 2016.

52. Geiger, J. as quoted at a meeting of the New York Metro Chapter of the Physicians for a National Health Program. New York, NY, June 14, 2016.

53. Ludwig, M. Resisting despair: Speaking truth in the face of Trump. *Truthout*, November 18, 2016.

54. Gilbert, G. Countering Trump: Let's build a people-powered democracy and economy. *Truthout*, November 19, 2016.

55. Potter, W, Penniman, N. *Nation on the Take: How Big Money Corrupts Our Democracy and What We Can Do About It*. New York. *Bloomsbury Press*, 2016, p. 228.

56. Jefferson, T. as quoted by Hightower, J, *The Hightower Lowdown*,18 (7): 1, July 2016.

57. Smith, H. The untold story of campaign 2016. *Reclaim the American Dream Blog*, June 21, 2016.

58. Republican support for single-payer. *Gallup poll*, May 16, 2016.

59. Keith Ensminger, Kramer Translation, Merced, CA. Personal communication, September 8, 2016.

60. Rmuse. GOP prohibits CBO from reporting how much ACA repeal blows up the deficit. *politicususa.com*, January 11, 2017.

61. Rovner J. Budget scorekeepers say GOP plan would raise the number of uninsured by 32M. *Kaiser Health News*, January 17, 2017.

62. McAuly, L. GOP doesn't want public to know how much Obamacare repeal will cost. Study shows it could be trillions. *Common Dreams*, January 7, 2017.

63. Reich, R. Once elected, Hillary must tap the power of Bernie's progressive movement. *The Progressive Populist*, September 15, 2016, p. 23.

64. *Indivisible: A Practical Guide for Resisting the Trump Agenda*. Available by contacting: indivisibleAgainstTrump@gmail.com

65. Smith, H. Can the states save American democracy? *Reclaim the American Dream Blog*, August 26, 2016.

66. Hightower, J. *The Hightower Lowdown*, November, 2016, p. 4.

67. Hacker, JS, Pierson, P. *American Amnesia: How the War on Government Led Us to Forget What Made America Prosper*. New York. *Simon & Schuster*. 2016, p. 338.

68. Gaffney, A, Woolhandler, S. Angell, M et al. Moving forward from the Affordable Care Act to a single-payer system. *Amer J Public Health* 106 (6): 987-988, June 2016.

69. Bauchner, H. Health care in the United States: A right or a privilege. *JAMA* 317 (1): 323, January 3, 2017.

70. Young, Q. *Everybody In Nobody Out: Memoirs of a Rebel Without a Pause*. Friday Harbor, WA. *Copernicus Healthcare*, 2013, pp. 239, 242.

Index

B

D

George Washington University, Milken School of Public Health, conclusions on APA repeal, 334

Georgia, insurance increases for individual health plans, 79

Gilead, marketing of Sovaldi, 46, 158

Gimlett, Dr. David, on San Juans, 237

Giroux, Henry, perspective on 2016 election, 320

GOP. *See* Republicans

Grob, Gerald, Rutgers, summary of mental health history, 167–168

Guttmacher Institute, report on historic low of abortion, 149

H

Hacker, Jacob (*American Amnesia*), 272–273, 291–292, 336–337

Hastings Center (*Goals of Medicine*), 297–298 (Table 22.1)

Harvard

    Dr. Francis Peabody talk, 117

    estimates of deaths/year from lack of health insurance, 98

Hayek, Friedrich A., economist, quote, 281

health care. *See also* ethical transformation; technical advances; U.S. health care

    administrative waste, 88, 301

    adverse impacts on physicians, 14

    as basic human right, 288, 293, 299

    "business ethic"/corporatized, 124

    as commodity, 115

    comparison with Canada as percentage of GDP (Fig. 6.1), 76, 78

    comparison of costs to other countries, 18, 70–71, 88

    competition, 281, 282

    cost-containment unsuccessful, 87

    costs

        paid by government (64 percent), 18

        rising in U.S.

        unaffordable/uncontrolled escalation, 261–262, 301

    debate, non-partisan, 299

    drug industry expenditures, 46

    failure at cost control, 87

    financing alternatives and reform, 301–302

    for-profit industry, 29 (Fig. 2.2), 87, 132

    high in 2016, 76

    high-deductible, increase, 328

    inflation beginning in 1965, 94

    instability of coverage, 68

    investor-owned firms, 129

I

N

S

Y

About the Author

John Geyman, M.D. is professor emeritus of family medicine at the University of Washington School of Medicine in Seattle, where he served as Chairman of the Department of Family Medicine from 1976 to 1990. As a family physician with over 21 years in academic medicine, he also practiced in rural communities for 13 years. He was the founding editor of *The Journal of Family Practice* (1973 to 1990) and the editor of *The Journal of the American Board of Family Medicine* from 1990 to 2003. Since 1990 he has been involved with research and writing on health policy and health care reform.

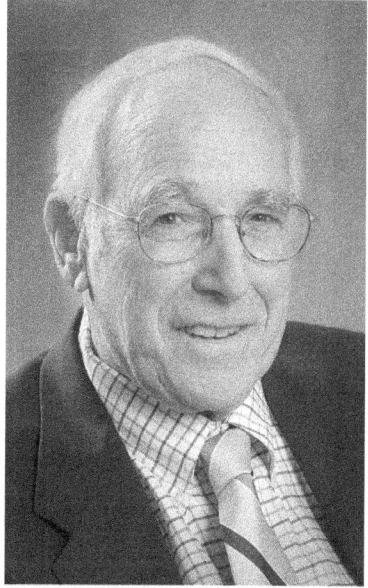

His most recent book was *The Human Face of ObamaCare: Promises vs. Reality and What Comes Next, How Obamacare Is Unsustainable: Why We Need a Single-Payer Solution For All Americans* (2015). Earlier books include *Health Care Wars: How Market Ideology and Corporate Power Are Killing Americans* (2012), *Souls On a Walk: An Enduring Love Story Unbroken by Alzheimer's* (2012), *Breaking Point: How the Primary Care Crisis Threatens the Lives of Americans* (2011), *Hijacked: The Road to Single Payer in the Aftermath of Stolen Health Care Reform (2010), The Cancer Generation: Baby Boomers Facing a Perfect Storm* (2009), *Do Not*

Resuscitate: Why the Health Insurance Industry Is Dying (2008), *The Corrosion of Medicine: Can the Profession Reclaim Its Moral Legacy* (2008), *Shredding the Social Contract: The Privatization of Medicare* (2006), *Falling Through the Safety Net: Americans Without Health Insurance (2005), The Corporate Transformation of Health Care: Can the Public Interest Still Be Served? (2004),* and *Health Care in America: Can Our Ailing System Be Healed?* (2002).

He served as the president of Physicians for a National Health Program from 2005 to 2007, and is a member of the National Academy of Medicine.